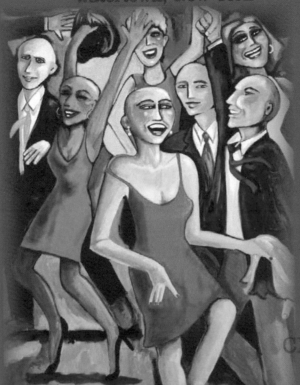

If Your Hair Falls Out, Keep Dancing!

How to cope with alopecia areata in a hair-obsessed world

Written and Illustrated by LeslieAnn Butler

©Nightengale Press
A Nightengale Media LLC Company

IF YOUR HAIR FALLS OUT, KEEP DANCING

For information about Nightengale Press please
visit our website at www.nightengalepress.com.
Email: publisher@nightengalepress.biz
or send a letter to:
Nightengale Press
10936 N. Port Washington Road. Suite 206
Mequon, WI 53092

Library of Congress Cataloging-in-Publication Data

Butler, LeslieAnn,
If You Hair Falls Out, Keep Dancing / LeslieAnn Butler
ISBN:1-933449-58-6
ISBN 13: 978-1933449-58-6
Health/Mind and Body

Copyright Registered: 2008
First Published by Nightengale Press in the USA

August 2008

10 9 8 7 6 5 4 3 2 1

Printed in the USA and the UK

Your hair is falling out.

You've just been told that the condition you have is called "alopecia areata." You might be thinking how this is the worst thing that's ever happened to you. Or maybe it's just one big inconvenience. Odds are, you're asking yourself, "Why me?"

"Why" may not be what you learn as you read *If Your Hair Falls Out, Keep Dancing!*, but you will find out what alopecia is and how to make the best of it.

LeslieAnn Butler, artist and writer, has experienced alopecia areata for more than thirty years. Here she offers stories and struggles of her own, and those of other women who have had alopecia in all its forms. Her experience, research and interviews have resulted in a book written in the voice of a good friend who wants to, and can, help. *If Your Hair Falls Out, Keep Dancing!* is filled with tips on how to tell your family and friends, available treatments, doctors, makeup, wigs, and most important, attitude.

If Your Hair Falls Out, Keep Dancing! is illustrated with LeslieAnn's colorful expressionist paintings that reflect her passion, humor and zest for life.

Perhaps you'll be inspired, find a pearl of wisdom, even have a laugh.

For sure, you'll find that you can enjoy and celebrate your life with alopecia areata, go after your dreams, and know you're not alone.

If Your Hair Falls Out, Keep Dancing! is not only for women with alopecia, but for their families and friends who would like a greater understanding of the condition.

*Posters of **Bald Boogie** (cover) are available from the National Alopecia Areata Foundation.*
All proceeds from the sales of the posters go to benefit NAAF.

What makes us different can also make us beautiful.

Lala Erlandson Butler, my mother

Acknowledgements

Thanks and great appreciation to the following: the lovely women who participated in our focus group in Portland, Oregon; Doctors Janet Roberts and Manuel Casanova; BK and Amber; and all my haired and hairless friends across North America and in England.

The First Dance

"I'm beautiful, I'm beautiful, I'm beautiful, dammit!
I'm beautiful, I'm beautiful, I'm beautiful, dammit!
...well, I woke up one morning, flossed my teeth, and decided,
'Damn, I'm fierce! (You look good)
You can be just like me (a goddess?!!) Yeah!
Don't just pussy foot around and sit on your assets.
Unleash your ferocity upon an unsuspecting world!
Rise and repeat after me: 'I'm beautiful!'
Ain't this my sun, ain't this my moon, ain't this my world,
To be who I choose!"

Lyrics from *I'm Beautiful,* written by Brinsley Evans,
sung by Bette Midler, CD "Bathhouse Betty"

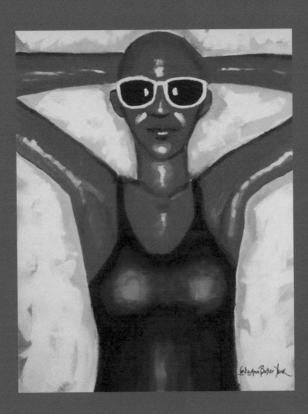

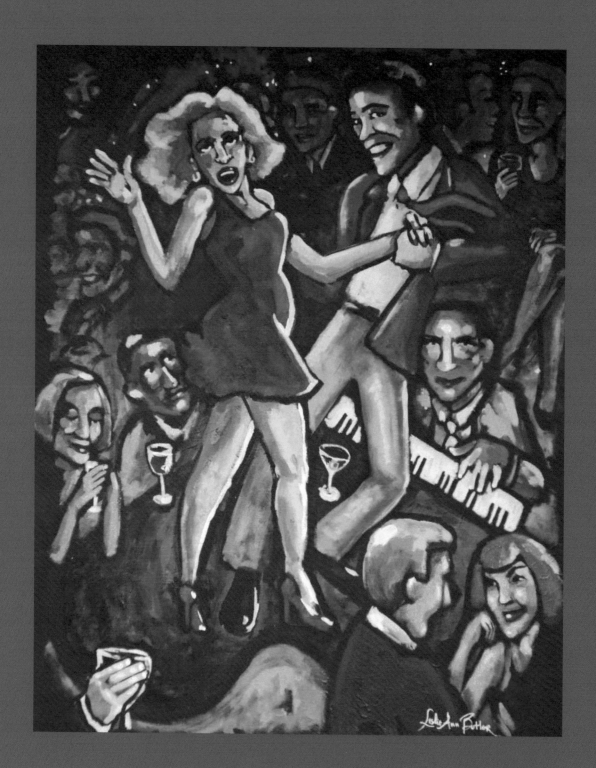

Preface

"Devil with the Blue Dress" is my song.

It all started at a now-defunct place to dance in Portland, Oregon called The Rafters. I was there almost every week and requested "Devil" every time. I loved to dance fast and never got tired of this song! Soon the DJ learned to watch for me, and the minute he spotted me walk through the door (before I even sat down!) he put the needle down on "Devil." On one particular night, my entrance was the same as usual: a choreography of throwing my coat and purse on the floor, waving to the DJ, gyrating my body to "good golly Miss Molly."

Except this time, I was in my wig. It was the first time I was going to attempt to rock and roll in my wig – held onto my perfectly bald head by a couple of measly pieces of tape.

I had thought long and hard about giving up fast dancing. With all those crazy moves, I was terrified that my fake hair would fly off into someone's gin and tonic.

But dancing was a part of me, and I finally got up the courage to go for it.

Because of Molly.

As I walked onto the floor that night, I heard the familiar words:

Fee, fee, fi, fi, fo-fo, fum
Look at Molly dance, here she comes
Wearin' her wig hat *and shades to match*
She's got high-heel shoes and an alligator hat. [1]

At that moment, I decided I wasn't going to let being bald and wearing a wig keep me from something I loved to do. Just like "Molly."

I tempted fate. I started dancing. Just like I used to, flipping my hair with wild abandon to the beat of the music.

No matter how much I threw my head around, my wig didn't come off.

I realized that if it did, well, what the hell.

And I kept right on dancing.

1 Lyrics from "Devil with the Blue Dress" by Mitch Riyder and and Detroit Wheels

Contents

Foreword

As a dermatologist specializing in the treatment of hair disorders, my path first crossed with LeslieAnn Butler's many years ago. She came to me searching for answers about this mysterious condition. Since then, our paths have continued to cross throughout the years. LeslieAnn is a special person with an amazing, "can do" attitude. *If Your Hair Falls Out, Keep Dancing! How to Cope with Alopecia Areata in a Hair-Obsessed World* is the result of her positive approach to life, her extensive research into this condition, and her determination to help other women with alopecia areata.

With humor and hope, *If Your Hair Falls Out, Keep Dancing!* takes alopecia areata out of the closet and exposes it to the bright light of day. This book is an excellent guide for women of all ages in any state of alopecia, for their families, friends and for their doctors.

I wish I could say that we have surefire treatments and proven answers. As yet, there's no cure. But medical science has come a long way in answering the "whys" of alopecia areata. And as science advances in the treatment of autoimmune disorders, we are moving much closer to the day when we will have effective treatments and eventually a cure.

Janet L. Roberts, MD
Physician and Surgeon
Dermatology Specialists Northwest
Member of the NAAF Scientific Advisory Council
Portland, Oregon

Introduction: Is Everyone Hairy Except Me?

For many people, having alopecia is the most difficult thing they've ever had to come to terms with.

Our society doesn't help.

Hair care is everywhere. People spend tens of millions of dollars to fluff, puff, shine, straighten, spike, curl, chunk, chop, grease, grow, tease, tousle, transplant, and otherwise clean, preen and keep the locks they have.

Women's magazines are filled with ads for products related to hair. Along with gowns, hairstyles are the first thing reporters recount and fashionistas study when they scan what celebrities are sporting.

And if they're not trying to beautify and keep the hair on their heads, they're trying to get rid of hair everywhere else. Shaving, tweezing, dissolving, waxing, annihilating stray hairs on toes, tummies, arms, chins, legs, bottoms.

And in this hair-obsessed society, I am totally bald. Everywhere.

Yep! No plucking my eyebrows, no slathering mascara on my eyelashes, no shaving my legs, no bikini waxes. I have alopecia universalis, the most severe form of this autoimmune disorder. And you know what? That's okay with me.

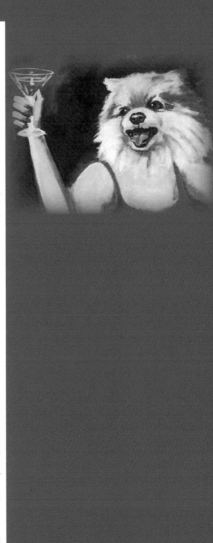

Hair Today, Gone Tomorrow

When I first lost my hair I felt isolated. Now I've lived with alopecia for over thirty years. Although now I accept it all – who I am and where I am on my journey – there are days I still long for and dream about having hair, and the more the better. What I wouldn't give for a bad hair day!

When you first encounter the fact of your alopecia, it's common to be overcome by fear, anger and depression. The future is uncertain; your life feels out of control. You are certain you are disfigured. And there's no guarantee that you will ever be "normal" again.

Whatever you do, the most important thing to remember is that your hair may come and go, and you will never know why it happened. You can't control it. It's not your diet or your stress level. It's not your fault. And it's not the end of the world.

Acceptance will come with time. But first we all go through a grieving process, because it is a "death" and a loss. After acceptance, thousands of women with AA lead a full and happy life, complete with husbands, boyfriends, children, good jobs and playing sports.

After all the struggling and sorting, I am doing just fine with it. In fact, it's often fun (yes, I know it's hard to believe – more about that later)! So I hope that by telling my story I might help other women how to find their own acceptance, self-confidence and style.

Sisters Under the Scalp

If Your Hair Falls Out, Keep Dancing! is devoted to my "follicular sisters," women and girls of all ages who have various types of alopecia for a variety of reasons. Women with small spots of baldness or total hairlessness, who are afraid, hopeless, angry, determined, coping. Women trying to live their lives around alopecia. Women who are doing well but need to know they're not alone. Women whose concerns are often ignored or trivialized. And why? Because alopecia areata isn't really a disease, or because it doesn't hurt or kill you. At least physically.

People with this condition are generally otherwise perfectly healthy. But emotionally, it can be terribly painful — and for some of us, the most traumatic experience we will ever go through. It can affect every aspect of your life. But alopecia areata doesn't have to have that much power. You will discover this as you meet the numerous wonderful women who have generously and unselfconsciously shared with me their sorrows, their depressions, their fears and funny stories, as well as their opinions on what has helped them come to terms with alopecia areata. I've learned something from each and every one of them, and I'm sure you will, too.

These brave women come from all over the world. Some I met in a focus group that Dr. Janet Roberts and I held in my home. Many, on line who found my name on the NAAF website as they were looking for help with their newly-discovered condition. Others on Dr. Manuel Casanova's web postings. And some through friends of friends.

(Although this book is for ladies, I want to acknowledge that alopecia is as emotionally upsetting to men as it is to women – sometimes even more so.

Women can wear wigs, eye makeup and false eyelashes. Aside from donning wigs or hairpieces, most men aren't going to be caught dead anywhere with eye makeup! So while it may be very cool to sport a bald or shaven head today, male alopecia sufferers still have to face the world with no eyebrows, eyelashes or body hair.)

Included are stories and quotes from Laura, a realtor who is newly single and newly balding; Nicole, a married sales representative and horsewoman; Kathy, who has a partner of twenty years and a son, and is working as an account administrator in an insurance agency; Karen, married with no children, a charity fund raiser; Paula, a business owner whose daughter and niece also have alopecia; Julie, a single physical therapist; Natasha, a young, married teacher with a baby daughter; Liz, who doesn't have alopecia, but her daughter just recently began to lose her hair at age twelve; Belinda, nineteen, who started losing her hair at age nine; Hannah, a college student who has had alopecia since she was four years old, and many, many more.

As you read their stories, you will realize you are not alone. You are part of a community of thousands of capable, self-assured, healthy women who are redefining themselves, embracing their femininity, and discovering their inner power and spiritual strength through coping with alopecia areata.

AA can be a catalyst for positive change, strengthening ourselves from within, and finding our hearts open to more than we ever had before. I can almost guarantee that one day you will look in the mirror and like the woman you see. You might even tell her, "Hello, Beautiful!" Meanwhile, you are creating a new relationship with yourself. And don't worry if it doesn't happen overnight.

So while you can't grow hair, alopecia areata brings a great opportunity for other kinds of growth. You have the choice and the power. And a lot of other women to support you.

I hope you enjoy reading *If Your Hair Falls Out, Keep Dancing*. And I wish you the very best. Please always remember that beauty isn't what's on your head, it's what's in your heart.

And keep dancing!

Hey, believe me. Baldness will catch on. When the aliens come, who do you think they're gonna relate to?

— George Costanza, Seinfeld character

Endorsements

"This "how-to" book provides a much needed text on dealing with emotional and cosmetic aspects of hair loss, whether from alopecia areata or chemotherapy. It details where to find and how to use products for compensating with this loss. It is written in the same bold and bright style that characterizes LeslieAnn's illustrations." —*Janet Roberts, M.D., Portland OR*

"A great read. It's like 'Sex and the City meets alopecia areata!'" —*Ann Wall Frank, Author*

"Many of my patients lose their hair from chemotherapy. This book will be as valuable a resource for them as it is for those with other conditions. The author touches with sensitivity and humor on the grief and self image issues that women face with hair loss—and her own triumphs create a positive path for others to deal with these issues. It's full of advice that cannot be found anywhere else but in the hands of someone who has been down this road. The paintings make this a literal work of art and add immeasurably to the book. Extraordinary." —*Joanna M. Cain, M.D., Oregon Health and Science University*

"This book is helpful, hopeful, funny and fabulous. It's full of practical advice about wigs, intimate encounters, the inappropriate questions from strangers, and other issues you face when every day is a bad hair day. Women with alopecia, LeslieAnn Butler is your new best friend!" —*Margie Boulé, Columnist, The Oregonian*

"... warm, engaging and sometimes downright hilarious, LeslieAnn offers advice to women dealing with a devastating condition. A must-have for anyone diagnosed with alopecia areata!" —*Mary Jane Horton, Horton & Gregory Associates Literary Agency, Los Angeles*

"Being a parent with a daughter who has alopecia areata, I thoroughly enjoyed reading this book. It provides as information-rich, practical, indispensable and entertaining "how to" guide for women and girls affected by this condition. I can't wait for my daughter to read it, too." —*Manuel F. Casanova, M.D., University of Louisville*

"After years of hair loss, LeslieAnn has made herself transparent for those of us dealing with similar issues. She has put herself under the microscope to make our walk easier. Thank you Leslie Ann, for your help, your caring and your self exposure." —*Amber Humphrey, Amber's Anointed Touch Hair Replacement, Inc.*

"...an essential read, whether you've lost hair, or care about someone who has. Leave it to LeslieAnn to bring humor and glamour to a difficult topic. She is a living testament that the lack of flowing locks is no reason not to live your most glamorous and joyful life. Be inspired and uplifted by this remarkable woman's personal journey." —*Nita Lina Howard, Author of* **A Woman's Journey is Her Legacy**

"LeslieAnn Butler takes us on a journey through all aspects of a life-altering condition, imparting her knowledge, advice, humor, and most important, attitude. Everything about this fabulous book, from the illustrations to the anecdotes and quotes, is aimed at helping women and girls not just cope, but thrive." —*Julie K. Gottlieb, owner, Gottlieb Gallery, Portland, OR*

"A great book for anyone facing challenge or adversity." —*Brenda Kay, Owner, Brenda Kay Hair Specialties*

I never really liked hairy women.
— *Marlow Butler, my father*

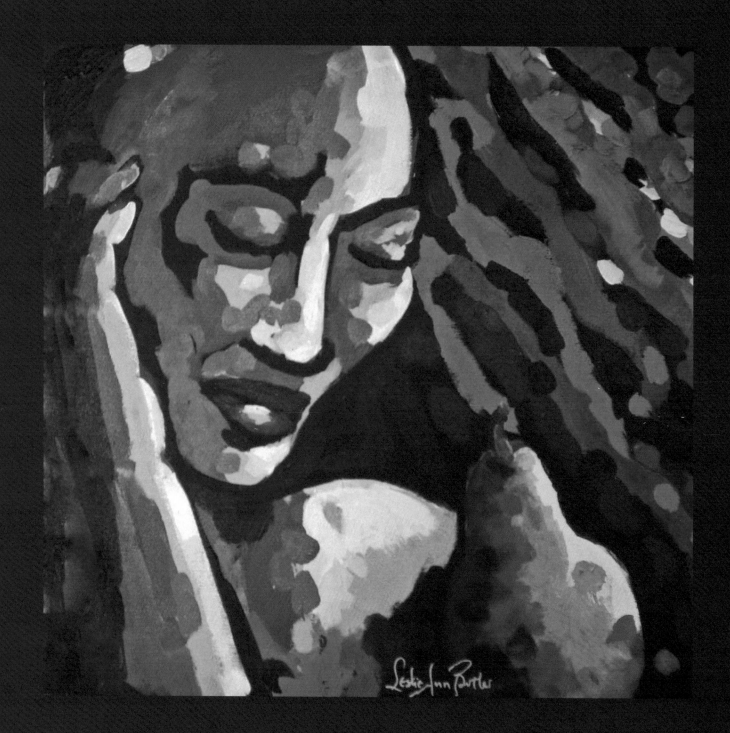
Leslie Ann Butler

CHAPTER ONE

Losing It

Once upon a time, I had a full, luxuriant head of hair.

It was about the time Charlie's Angels was a popular television show. Remember Farrah Fawcett? That feathered, golden mane made headlines. I copied the style. As funny as it may look today, big hair was in!

As I was getting ready for work, I noticed a small, round bald spot behind my ear. Instead of wearing my hair up that day as I had planned to, I wore it long and full and made a panicked appointment to the dermatologist.

"Was it an allergic condition," I asked? "Was it from brushing my hair too much? Pulling my pony tail too tight?" The doctor shrugged and told me that it was called alopecia areata, and was probably caused by stress. It's no big deal, he said, just take things easy. He started me on cortisone injections and sent me on my way.

As per the doctor's instructions, I did my best to chill out. I even got a prescription for sedatives. After taking one tablet, I slept for twenty-four hours. I couldn't think straight. That was the end of tranquillizers.

The cortisone injections encouraged my hair to grow back. At first soft and fuzzy like down, then my normal, thick mane. Whew, that's over, I thought.

But it happened again.

And again. In the same spot, in different spots. Bigger spots, smaller ones. All shapes and sizes. They reminded me of the animal-shaped pancakes my dad made me when I was a little kid. I wore my tires out driving back and forth to my doc's office for cortisone injections, panic attacks, comforting words. And all the while I tried not be stressed out, which in itself was very stressful.

After a number lectures about my stress levels, I finally decided that my doctor actually didn't know very much about alopecia areata. To his credit, he did know that there was no known cause and no cure (at least that part was true). It was different than male pattern baldness in that the hair falls out in patches, usually circular. He said there was nothing to do except the cortisone injections. At that time, that was also true. Although they were very painful, I thought they were worth it because my hair grew back in a predictable fashion.

I resigned myself to the possibility that my spotty spots would indefinitely continue to come and go, and come again. I camouflaged them by rubbing in dark blond eyebrow pencil. Wigs and falls were very trendy at the time, so I had a "wig wardrobe" — several different colors, lengths and styles. I worked part time in a wig shop so I could learn more about how to care for them.

Years passed and my hairstyles were totally dependant on the location and size of my latest spots. The alopecia slowly continued to get worse.

One morning as I was getting ready for the first day of my new job as creative director for an advertising agency, I was horrified to find that one bald spot had appeared in my right eyebrow, and another in the middle of a section of eyelashes. I burst into angry tears. Damn! Losing the majority of the hair on my head was bad, but manageable. Where before I had worn wigs and falls once in awhile when things got really bad, I was now wearing wigs full time. But how in the world could I possibly cope with having no eyelashes and eyebrows? I went to work red-eyed, depressed and cursing whatever twist of fate had brought me to this horrible state.

And a year or two later, it all—completely, everywhere—fell out. I was forty-one.

Some days I looked like a creature from outer space. Other days, I looked more like a doorknob.

I had heard that some insurance companies covered the cost of wigs, and decided to go for it. A "hair prosthesis" was what wig companies called them, to better encourage the insurance companies to pay. I wrote a comprehensive letter and sent them a photo of my bare head and face, and included a sad expression on my face.

They turned me down. A wig was a cosmetic, not medical, need they claimed. I guess the lack of eyebrows and eyelashes kept me from looking sad enough.

I continued my quest for answers: Maybe it wasn't stress, but perhaps a deficiency in my diet. I tried vitamins, herbs, and brackish nutritional drinks with unidentifiable ingredients. I tried high and low protein diets. I tried a yeast-free diet, a sugar-free diet, a caffeine-free diet, a food-free diet. I tried spreading smelly goos and sticky creams onto my scalp and wearing a plastic bag over the top so it would "cook in." I gave myself vigorous head rubs until my scalp was red and sore.

Or was it bad karma (maybe I was an Indian who had scalped one too many cowboys)? I tried hypnosis with several different hypnotists, including an unpleasant and somewhat smelly doctor who informed me I hated men, and a creepy man who worked out of his hotel room and told me my mother had drowned me in a past life and by the way, he thought I had beautiful lips. A psychic told me I used to live in ancient Egypt and everyone shaved their heads then, and I liked it that way, so there you have it.

One of them decided that maybe it was lack of sun, since I live in a rainy climate – so I went in for heat lamp treatments and sat in the sun bareheaded as much as possible. It didn't work, but I did get a sunburn and a few freckles on my scalp. Then I graduated to a frightening electronic device with blue lights that zapped my scalp with crackling noises, reminiscent of when they bring the dead back to life in those horror movie laboratories.

I flew to Los Angeles to receive "Shakti Pat" from an Eastern guru (a touch on the head). I'm not sure what that was, but everyone around me who received it seemed to be swooning in spiritual ecstasy. Unfortunately, all it did was make my nose run.

I listened night and day to subliminal healing tapes that provided whispering messages under the sounds of the ocean, and caused my co-workers to ask if there was something wrong with the plumbing in our office.

Life can be wildly tragic at times and I've had my share. But, whatever happens to you, you have to keep a slightly comic attitude. In the final analysis, you have got to not forget to laugh.

Katharine Hepburn

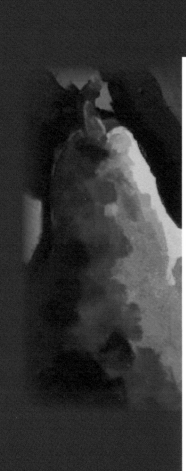

I tried greasy castor oil packs that ruined my brand new sheets.

I visualized myself with all my hair back. I tried positive affirmations like, "I am now covered in hair." (I figured too much hair would be better than too little!) I filled four yellow tablets with the words, "My hair is now growing back completely. I have a full, healthy head of hair." All I got was writer's cramp.

Why did nothing work, I furiously demanded, shaking my fists heavenward? I was angry and astounded that there was no cure, no answer, and very little knowledge about this mysterious condition. My world was out of control. I really wanted to know why. Why? *Why meeeeee???*

I grieved. I cried. I prayed. I gnashed my teeth. I lamented, "What have I done to deserve this?" Maybe I *had* scalped cowboys.

I hated wearing a wig. It itched, it was hot. It came off when I didn't want it to. So the next question I asked myself was, could I blithely run around sans wig and declare my freedom from hair? No, no matter how adorable Sinead O'Connor was, or that Sigourney Weaver had shaved her head for "Alien," (so how come she didn't *look* like one?) I still thought I looked like a doorknob. Would I ever be willing and able to casually show anyone my head except my doctor? Absolutely not. I'd rather show my undies in public than my my baldness.

Hoping for some new answers, I went to an AA (alopecia areata) support group here in Portland, headed up by renowned dermatologist Janet Roberts, MD. Only women were there. Their stories would have made my hair stand on end, if I'd had any.

One young woman had practically become a recluse, going out in public only if it was extremely important (for example, if her house caught on fire). Another wept because her husband had left her when she lost her hair. A third woman was angry at her situation and had quite the chip on her shoulder. She used a lot of four-letter words.

There were several others, but the point was that I didn't identify with anyone in the group. I had actually begun to feel bit a little guilty about wanting my hair back again. "I refuse to be a crybaby! I could be in a lot worse shape," I thought. "I'm perfectly healthy in every other way. It's not like the condition is life-threatening. Just very, very inconvenient." I was coping just fine. "Who needs a support group?" I thought. I didn't go back.

I didn't really talk about my condition except to people who were very close to me. Men who I was getting cozy with, who I knew were going to touch my hair; a woman friend who pulled on a long black hair in the midst of my blonde (fake) mane; a friend who spotted some wefting.

I became very involved in charity work. My painting career took off. My first book was published. I had wonderful friends and my life was terrific. I thought, "I finally have it together." All of a sudden, I realized that even without hair, I was happier and more grateful than I had ever been. And the idea for this book was born.

Now it's your turn to go forward. With some adjustments to the inconvenience, a few little makeup tricks, good hair augmentation and the right attitude, you can live with alopecia areata. And live well.

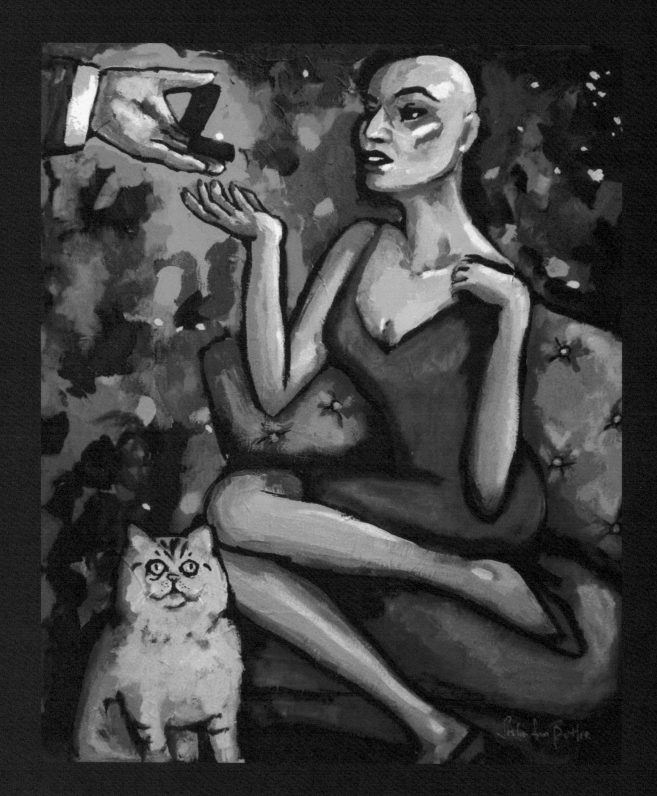

CHAPTER TWO

What the heck is this?

It's not a disease. That's the good news.

It's not catching, and it doesn't destroy the hair follicles. And interestingly, as reported by the National Alopecia Areata Foundation, AA is as common as psoriasis, affecting nearly five million people in the United States alone. It affects men and women of all races and all age groups equally. Approximately 60% of alopecia sufferers develop this condition before the age of twenty.

Technically, alopecia areata (the umbrella term for patchy to total hair loss) is an auto-immune disorder – like arthritis, eczema, or asthma. The body's T-cells (white cells found in lymph nodes, bone marrow and blood) identify hair follicle cells as invaders and attack them. (How come our autoimmune systems are so dumb?) Normal scalp hair processes through three phases: growth, degeneration, and resting (when the hair falls out). This process is staggered on the scalp. With alopecia areata, all the hair in one section will enter the degeneration phase at the same time, resulting in patchy bald spots or total baldness. The follicles are not destroyed – just dormant. Of all alopecia sufferers, only about 2% of us have alopecia totalis (no head or facial hair), and universalis (no hair anywhere).

Typically, the first symptom is a little round bald spot, about the size of a quarter. Most of the time, it grows back. If you're lucky, that's the end of it! I'm amazed at the large number of women I know who have had alopecia temporarily – after a few weeks it goes away, never to bother them again. Others have patchy spots that come and go.

For me and a number of other women, alopecia areata has progressed over the years. At first it was just a small spot which went away. Later the spots became bigger. Some stayed and some filled in. About fourteen years after my first episode with this condition, all my hair fell out including eyelashes and eyebrows. Losing my eyelashes and eyebrows was the worst.

"Now I look like a mask! I could rent my face out for Halloween!" says Julie, twenty-eight, a physical therapist. "I have absolutely no facial expression until I paint on my eyes and brows. And the worst part is that I still have hair on my *toes*!"

Nicole thinks she looks like an alien. "I can't look at myself in the mirror without hair. It's too awful."

Obviously, alopecia is not fair. I, too, sometimes will find a few hairs on my toes, and one chin hair pops out now and then. Ugh! I dispatch those immediately. But there are one or two lone hairs – like a beloved single pale brown one in my eyebrow area – that, even though they serve no purpose, I want to keep (as a symbol of hope, I suppose). Laura, a forty-year-old realtor, says, " I have only a couple of small tufts of hair on my head, but I can't bring myself to shave it yet! It would be admitting defeat."

So what causes alopecia? No one really knows. Stress has not been proven to be the cause, although stress can impair immune system functioning. It's most likely that alopecia areata develops as a consequence of a combination of external and genetic causes. The most current research points to the possibility of a strong genetic link in many cases. For example, those who develop alopecia areata for the first time after age thirty are less likely to have another family member with it. If patches first occur before thirty, it's probably hereditary. And speaking of heredity, if you are worried about passing the gene on to your children you can be comforted with the fact that experts report there is only a 7% chance of that. Those are great odds!

According to *When a Woman Goes Bald,* an article by Barry Yeoman in the February 2006 issue of Discover Magazine, geneticists have begun finding clues that may eventually lead to treatment for alopecia. One woman in particular, Angela Christiano, a molecular geneticist at Columbia University in New York City, is particularly interested in pinning down the mutations that cause alopecia areata, because she has also been affected: alopecia areata, totalis and universalis run in Christiano's family. Currently, she is finding clusters of susceptibility genes. The fact that the research is going on and that one of the researchers is a "sister under the scalp," makes me feel pretty positive about the future!

Baldness is still relatively rare in women, and is generally treated as as sign of crisis or stress—or...a sign of madness.

Patrick Barham, Journalist

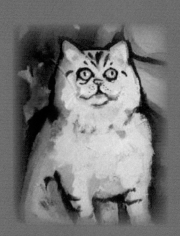

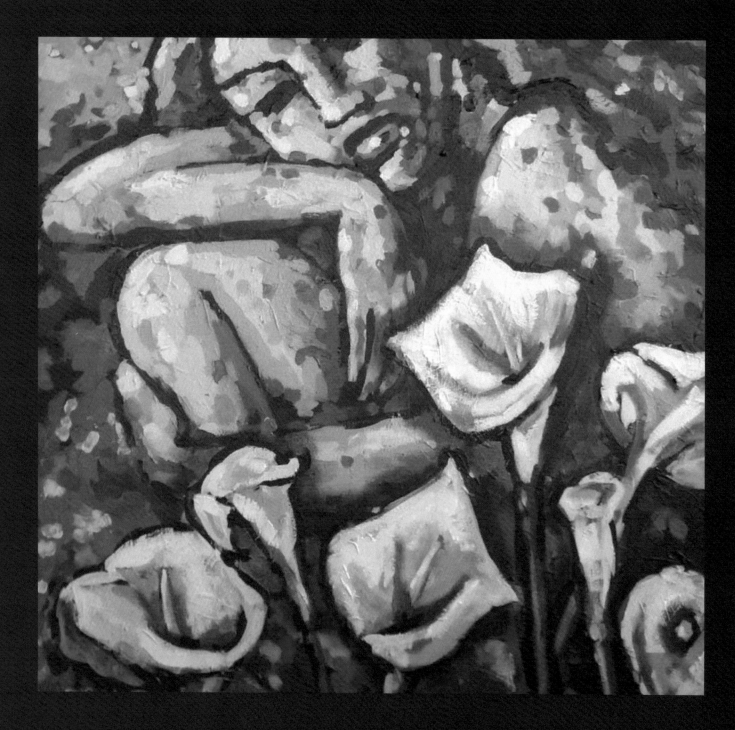

CHAPTER THREE

Nights of a Thousand Tears

The loss of your hair is different from other losses.

It's not considered a true handicap like the loss of a leg, a finger, an eye. People may be fearful when they see patchy hair, thinking it's a fatal or contagious condition. But alopecia is the very visible loss of a function of your body. And coping with baldness is just as difficult as coping with another bodily loss.

Anything that changes the way you look on the outside will affect how you feel on the inside. So of course you will grieve. And it's all right; it's normal. You can show the outside world your stiff upper lip, but then you can come home and cry. We all have.

"I always depended on my looks to get by," Laura told me. "Then two years ago my hair began to fall out. Every morning I had to gather it up off the bathroom floor and the shower drain and throw it away. I thought I looked horrible. I refused to be photographed. I didn't wear a wig because I thought somehow everyone would be able to tell. I cried a thousand tears. I woke up every night in a cold sweat, hoping it was just a bad dream. To say I was depressed is an understatement. I was angry, embarrassed, ashamed. I lashed out at people; my work suffered, my relationships suffered. I drank too much to try to kill the pain. I ranted and raved, 'Why me?' I felt totally out of control. I thought, 'Who will be able to love me now that I am like this?'" (By the way, Laura is now happily dating a wonderful guy who doesn't care at all how much or how little hair she has.)

Like any other kind of grief, discovering alopecia can shut you down. When she realized she actually could lose all her hair, Julie couldn't eat or sleep. "When my coworkers began to notice how thin I had become, I decided I'd better do something, and I joined a support group. Most of the women there were crying, just like me. It helped me see that it wasn't shallow to feel bad about losing my hair."

Nicole says she still grieves from time to time. "Sometimes I don't feel like going out in public at all – I just want to lock myself away. But since I can't live like that, I try to surround myself with people who like me, hair or no hair! Sometimes I dream I have hair again – I'm on a roller coaster, with my long blonde hair streaming out behind me in the wind. Then my cat licks my bald head in the morning and wakes me up."

"One minute I'm doing okay, and I think I can handle it," says Caroline, a thirty-year-old writer. "Then, the smallest thing can set me back. I can't imagine having to deal with alopecia for the rest of my life. I have to believe it will somehow go away or be cured."

"The worst thing is the whole dating business," says Julie. "I hate flinching when a new man reaches for my hair. I am so full of anger about having to constantly explain this horrible disorder to everyone, and tired of being embarrassed about it! It's so unfair! For so long I have tried to accept it, and I've come a long way – but I still feel angry, ashamed, and I still cry."

Paula, a forty-eight-year-old business owner, has battled alopecia areata since she was twenty-four and says that she continues to be 'in denial.' "Most often I here people talk about 'denial' as if it was a bad thing," she says. "But having a certain sense of denial about my own alopecia has been a great coping mechanism. By this, I am referring to my way of not looking for new spots, not noticing if my hair is no longer thick and lovely, not dwelling on my condition. After all, intellectually speaking, life is about much more than hair. Yet if I let my 'denial guard' down, the pain of this gets to me."

Kathy, a thirty-nine-year-old account administrator, had a meltdown in the parking lot on the way out of her dermatologist's office. "I had just received some injections and was supposed to go back for more in a month. I was sure I'd be completely bald by then! I cried so hard I couldn't drive myself home and had to get my mom to come and get me."

She called in sick to work. "I loved my hair, and it turned on me. I felt out of control and horribly betrayed."

After being treated with cortisone-derivative shots for her bald spots, Angela Christiano, PhD, a molecular geneticist at Columbia University in New York City, lived in perpetual fear: "You wake up every morning and before you lift your head off the pillow, you think, 'Is it all there? Is it gone?' And then you get angry at yourself for being so vain. I thought, 'I just spend five years working on lethal skin diseases. I should count my blessings that this is all I have.' And that doesn't work."(*When a Woman Goes Bald,* Discover Magazine, February 2006)

"I feel trapped," says Julie. "I can't go outside and work in the yard anymore because my wig is so itchy and hot. I don't want to work out at my health club because I will sweat in this wig. I'm scared my children might get this. I go through bouts of terrible sadness. Then I feel guilty because after all, it's just hair. People tell me I'm lucky I don't have something worse. That makes me feel horribly shallow. Is there something wrong with me for feeling this way?"

Ashely Siegel, cofounder of the National Alopecia Areata Foundation, writes about her experience as she tried to cope:

"The effect alopecia areata seems to have on people is to wipe out their self-esteem in a matter of moments. The whole ordeal from the dermatologist's office to the wig salon is often one degrading experience after another. Feeling so helpless and vulnerable, we wander around 'inside out' until we can put the pieces together again. I pushed people away for years. I missed out on feeling good and having great relationships for too long. I was afraid of the wind, of sex, of having people too close to my face. I suspected that everyone told their friends about me and when I passed them on the street they said, 'Oh, there's Ashely Siegel, the one with no hair.'" *(NAAF Newsletter no. 41, September/ October 1989)*

We all go through this. It's a natural process. You aren't alone in your anger, fear, vulnerability, depression. It's a natural process, and you have to go through it. We all do.

The good news is that by allowing yourself to grieve over your loss, you will come to terms with it by working through grief's natural stages of denial, anger, depression,

When one door of happiness closes, another opens; but often we look so long at the closed door that we do not see the one which has opened for us.

Helen Keller

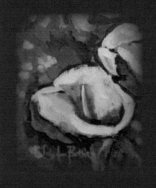

bargaining and acceptance. Sooner or later, you will arrive at acceptance – *yes, you will get there*, sometimes with a little or a lot of outside help – empowering you to begin living a fulfilling life with a renewed sense of self. For help, a support group can be wonderful. To find one in your community, contact the National Alopecia Areata Foundation or your dermatologist who is familiar with alopecia areata. Professional counseling can also be beneficial as a safe place to explore your feelings and work out your fears and concerns.

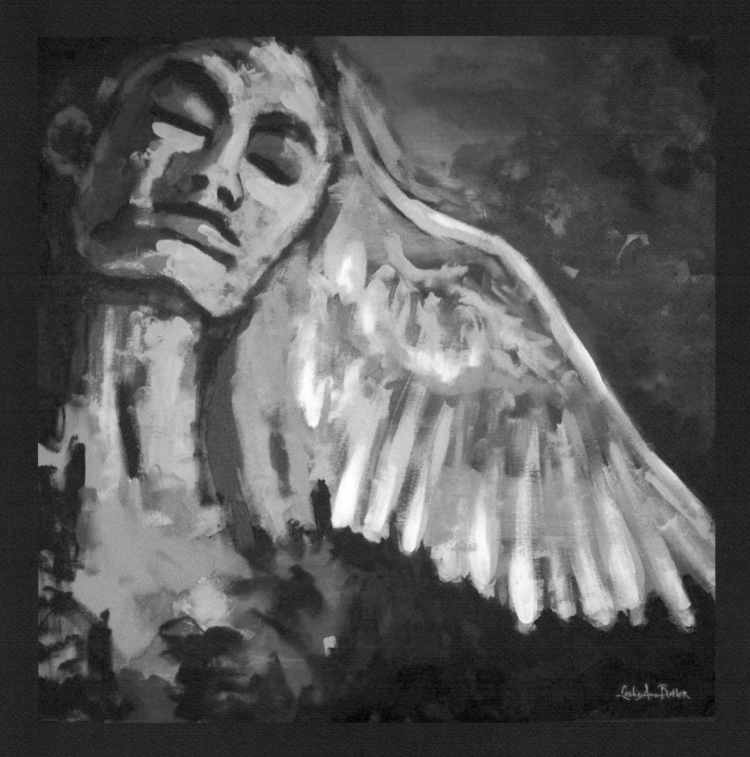

CHAPTER FOUR

Dealing with Doctors and Drugs

"There's not much we can do. You'll just have to live with it."

"It's caused by stress. Lighten up."

"Your hair will probably grow back. And if it doesn't – well, at least be thankful alopecia areata isn't gonna kill you!"

Some doctors don't have much of a " bedside manner" when dealing with alopecia.

Dermatologists are not all the same. Many have a real lack of knowledge and understanding about alopecia. There are many stories of women who seek out dermatologists only to find that they know *volumes* more than the docs do. Others are up on the latest treatments and research. You want to pick a doctor who has it all: knowledge of the condition and the latest treatments available, understanding and empathy for you, thoroughness (for example, who asks about family history), and a healthy and supportive attitude.

Kathy has this story: "My HMO required that I go to a primary care physician to get a dermatologist referral. When I showed him my bald spot and asked for my referral, he refused! He told me to go home and forget about it, because you couldn't even see the spot unless you lifted my hair!"

32

Hannah, an art history student, told me that her parents took her to a naturopath when they discovered her alopecia. "That person didn't know much about alopecia areata; she said my condition was due to stress. That was a little hard to believe, seeing as how I was only four years old!"

For years, I went to doctor after doctor to find a "cure" for my condition. But now I don't bother because my alopecia is too severe. For my form of alopecia, docs can't do much of anything...at least, not yet. For milder forms there are treatments that can help, like cortisone injections into the hairless spots to blunt the immune-cell attack which will make the hair grow back temporarily. I even had injections in my eyebrow area, and my eyebrows grew back (a lot thinner than they were naturally). But besides giving me a lot of pain, the injections gave me what I call "Neanderthal Brow," big bumps that made me look like I was related to The Missing Link. (Fortunately, it went away a few months after I stopped the injections.)

The fact is, there's no cure for alopecia areata right now. There are some effective treatments; whether or not they will help depends on the severity of your alopecia. There is a very good chance that within a year or two, your hair will grow back completely with no medical help. For others including me, nothing has worked. If it does for you, fabulous! I envy you. What I have decided to do for myself is accept my lemons and make margaritas out of them, until they find a treatment that really works. Why put myself through the torture (let alone the money flying out the window) of needles, itchy ointments, pulsing light, or chanting while I drink eye of newt and powdered toad (after all, I am a vegetarian)?

There are two categories of treatments offered at this time, depending on the severity of the condition. Most responsive to treatment is when your alopecia is mild, with patchy spots and 50% or less of your hair is lost.

For mild alopecia, current available treatments include:

Cortisone Injections

This is the most common treatment, and the success rate is approximately 70%. Injections are made in the skin in and around the bald patches, and repeated every four to six weeks. If new hair grows in, it usually appears within six weeks. This treatment

There are 40 advantages of alopecia, including the fact that without hair you cannot get lice or get bats caught in your hair...

Kevin Baldwin, author

doesn't prevent new patches from appearing. Injections can be given in the eyebrow and eyelid areas as well as in the scalp. Occasionally, indentations or bumps will appear which are temporary and go away when treatment is discontinued.

Topical Minoxidil

Applied twice daily, a 5% minoxidil solution may grow hair in scalp and eyebrows. This is a safe, easy treatment. This works better for small patchy spots, but may also be tried for people who have more extensive loss (generally a 14% success rate for people with extensive alopecia areata or 75% to 90% hair loss). New growth will be noticed within three months and full regrowth in sixty-two weeks. For people with 100% hair loss or who have had alopecia areata for ten years or more, minoxidil probably won't help.

Combination Minoxidil and Cortisone Cream

By combining minoxidil with a topically-applied cortisone cream, results are often better than using either alone, with success rates as high as 50%. New hair growth can appear within three months.

Anthralin Cream or Ointment

Anthralin, applied to bare patches and left on long enough to cause minor itching and redness, increases the metabolic activity in the area it is used. It causes a reddish burn which can be painful. Again, the results have been mixed; if new hair appears, it is usually seen within twelve weeks. The cream will stain clothing and sheets, and care must be taken not to get it into the eyes.

For extensive alopecia areata where 50% or more of your hair is gone, there are different treatments:

Cortisone Pills

Taken internally, cortisone is much stronger than scalp injections. Although healthy young adults may tolerate cortisone pills well, there are side effects including a compromised immune system, which should be discussed with your doctor. Prolonged use is not recommended, and after pills are discontinued your regrown hair is likely to fall out again.

Topical Immunotherapy

Chemicals, like squaric acid dibutyl ester (SABDE) and diphenylcyclopropenone (DPCP), are applied to the hair loss areas. This produces an allergic rash or dermatitis. It is highly irritating and makes your skin itch. Hair growing results are mixed. New growth will be evident after six months, and treatment has to continue to keep it growing in. You can experience blistering, hives and loss of pigmentation in the contact area, or you may have few side effects.

Puva

PUVA, or psoralens and UVA therapy, consists of ingestion or topical application of chemical compounds found in plants and exposure to ultraviolet light, two or three times a week. It has had varying degrees of success, but the relapse rate is very high. Side effects can include sunburn, skin inflammation, itching, dizziness and conjunctivitis of the eyes. Long-term effects (for treatments continued for longer than one year) include cataracts if proper eye protection isn't used, premature skin aging, and non-melanoma skin cancer.

These treatments can help some people. "I have received hydro-cortisone injections in my eyebrows and scalp since I was in the sixth grade," says Hannah. "They work for me. I still get injections every six weeks. I also have eyelashes now, since I've been having cortisone injections in that area as well. Hooray, bring on the mascara!"

It's good to know what to expect, and what others have gone through. Although some women have had good results, there are many who haven't:

"It was miserable," says Ann, forty-seven and a psychologist, of her trial with SABDE. "I got such a terrible, itchy, oozy rash on my head I couldn't wear my wig. I didn't get any results, and it actually removed some of the pigmentation from my skin so now I have white blotches." Dr. Janet Roberts says that this unfortunate incident is the result of overtreatment. Under the care of a skilled physician, this would never have happened.

June, thirty-two, a teacher says, "I tried PUVA for nearly a year. It didn't work for me – but my doc got new furniture for her waiting room."

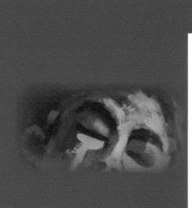

Bonnie, thirty-seven, mother of two says, "I only used Anthralin for five months. It was too much of a hassle. I had to smear it on twice a day, and it stained my clothes and sheets. It felt like a very bad sunburn. Did it work? No, but maybe I didn't give it enough time."

"After about five years of cortisone injections, I wound up with lumpy, stretched skin that hurt all the time. As soon as I stopped the shots, my hair fell out almost right away," says Tina, a realtor.

If you find that you have come to the point where you accept your condition and prefer not to get treatments, you're not alone.

"When I first found out I had alopecia areata," says Mary, forty-four, a printing rep," I went to my first alopecia support group with guns blazing, ready to travel to the ends of the earth and spend every last dime to find a cure or successful treatment. I couldn't believe how the other people in the group were just sitting there calmly, taking about wigs and makeup. I subsequently learned that they had been through my gung-ho stage and had reached acceptance of their condition."

Another example is Nicole who says that she has stopped treatments since her condition continued to get more severe. "I have gone from patchy bald spots on my head to losing all the hair on my head, plus eyelashes and eyebrows. For me, the treatments weren't doing any good and I was losing ground too fast."

Me too. I stopped pursuing treatment years ago. I won't try again until a cure is found. Let's hope that's soon! I have these visions of myself as a very old lady, drowsing in a rocking chair, not caring that my wig is on backwards. At least I won't have gray hair.

Voodoo and Other Miracle Cures

One of the worst treatments I heard of was from a woman whose doctor shaved a layer of skin off her scalp in the bald spots. Ouch! She grew scabs, but no hair. Another women tried vinegar rinses, and still another tried an old Latino treatment of cactus juice extract. She says, "What the heck; if nothing else it's a great hair conditioner!" But the prize goes to a man who was told by his dermatologist to put urine on his bald spots. In case you're wondering, it didn't work.

There are lots of people out there who would love to take your money for worthless "cures." Compost cream, shampoo made of horse saliva, eating twelve zucchinis a day

— these would work just as well as any of the "magic" cures, "guaranteed to grow hair" that abound. Nearly every "GROW HAIR!" product you see online, in magazines and infomercials is bogus. Don't waste your time or energy on the lure of false promises.

I know of no specially-formulated shampoos, oils or creams that will work. You can try all the vitamin therapy and homeopathic remedies if you wish, but I doubt if they will cure your alopecia. Neither will replacing silver fillings, sticking acupuncture needles into your scalp, getting colonics nor visualizing yourself covered with hair while chanting.

The best treatment is knowledge. Odds are, the more you know about alopecia areata, the more in control you will feel. My recommendation is to find out all you can about treatments, options, research, tips on cosmetics and wigs. I can almost guarantee that when you get a handle on this, you'll start to feel better.

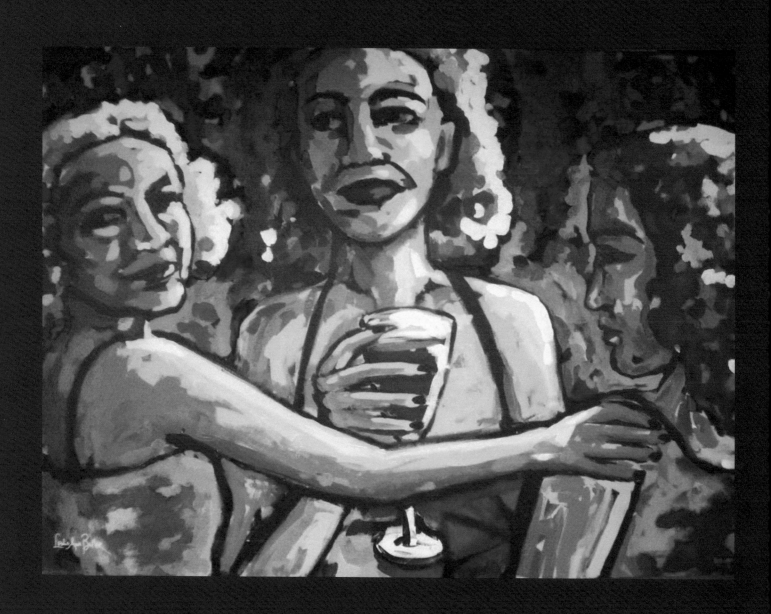

CHAPTER FIVE

Chemotherapy: Another Way to Lose Your Hair

Hair loss from chemotherapy is a completely different animal than alopecia areata. Although women who have chemo-related hair loss are practically guaranteed that their lovely locks will return, that doesn't make losing it any easier – at least at first. "The cancer didn't scare me. The surgery didn't scare me. But chemo scared the hell out of me! I cried when my oncologist told me I would lose my hair,"[1] said Leslie Moulton who was thirty-five years old when she discovered she had cancer. Medical experts say that some cancer patients even forego treatment for fear of the intense embarrassment that will result from the hair loss.[2]

Susan Dentzer, on-air correspondent with the Online News Hour, reports over a million Americans undergo chemotherapy for cancer each year. About half of them experience at least some hair loss. With chemotherapy, hair loss occurs because the drug targets all rapidly dividing cells – so healthy hair follicles, which are some of the fastest growing cells in the body, dividing every twenty-three to seventy-two hours, are destroyed along with the cancer cells. Within a few weeks after the first treatment, your hair begins to fall out – either gradually or dramatically. (Of course, not every woman experiences hair loss on chemotherapy. It depends on the drugs being used. That is something you can discuss with your physician.)

[1] *The Breast Cancer Book of Strength and Courage* by Ernie Bodai, M.D.
[2] News Hour with Jim Lehrer, January 8, 2001

Many women have told me that the worst part about chemo hair loss is the fact that it is a highly visible symbol of their illness. Karen, fifty-five, active in charity fundraising, told me that when she found out she had to have chemotherapy, the first thing she asked was if she would lose her hair. "I couldn't handle the thought that everyone would know that I was sick. It's one thing to be fighting a life-threatening disease, but then to have it be obvious to the world because I don't have hair – that's hard." Jackie, a forty-three -year -old old yoga instructor, said, "When I looked in the mirror, it was a constant reminder that something was seriously wrong."

To prepare themselves, many women cut their hair comfortably shorter. It's easier going from short to bald than from long to bald. It also lessens the shock of seeing lots of long hair everywhere as it's falling out.

I suggest looking for wigs while you still have hair so you can find a good color match. Another suggestion is to cut small sections of your hair in different places (top, sides and underneath, since your hair contains different shades), and put them separately in envelopes or plastic bags. Take them with you when you look for wigs and hair pieces. You can also have someone take a photo of you in your favorite hairstyle, which will help your wig stylist match it.

A lot of women found the challenge something they could cope with – even have fun with. Forty-year-old Mary, an architect, shared this: " I'd always wanted to be a blonde, so I bought a long, blonde wig. I liked it so much that after it grew back, I changed my own hair color to blonde."

One woman told me, "Within four weeks I lost all the hair on my head including eyelashes and eyebrows, and a majority of body hair. I got a really good wig. It was beautiful, and people said I looked ten years younger!"

Karen bought a wig early on. "I decided I would buy the best-looking wig I could find and have it ready. It was almost exactly like my own hair, but more beautiful – and no one could tell it wasn't real. For the first time in my adult life, I didn't have to worry about roots!"

Some women don't bother with wigs. Diana, fifty-one, refused to wear one. "I wore scarves and caps in every different color and style. Actually, that was fun. Even though I had no hair, I was able to live with it. And I knew it would grow back."

Martine, a corporate VP at thirty-five, said since she knew her hair would grow back, she decided to wear a scarf. "I wore beautiful scarves tied in creative ways and earrings, and I felt really good about myself. At night I wear a turban to keep my head warm."

Wigging It

If you decide you just can't do without hair, then a wig is for you. What kind should you get? Since your hair loss is almost always temporary, that may mean you would be happier buying a less expensive synthetic wig, which can last for several months, rather than a human hair piece which has a much longer life but can cost two to three thousand dollars. To help you make your decision, look at the information in Chapter Nine on wigs, scarves and other headcoverings.

...I've learned the hard way that...life is about not knowing, having to change, taking the moment and making the best of it without knowing what's going to happen next.

Gilda Radner

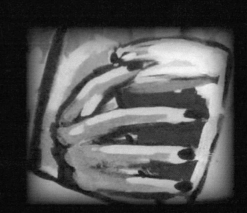

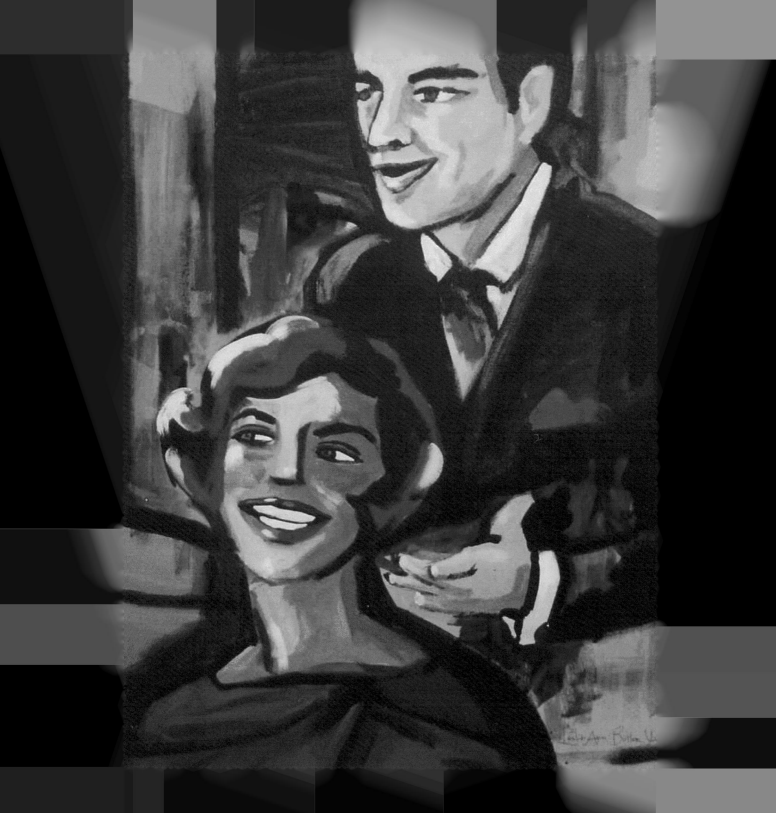

CHAPTER SIX

Pulling It Off

Only Your Hairdresser Knows for Sure

When I first discovered I had alopecia, I was in my twenties and dating a man who watched the spots come and go with me. He was wonderful about it. We eventually married. Then he developed cancer and died within a year. We both experienced hair loss: him by chemo, me by alopecia. After going through that, I realized even more that my disorder was nothing compared to what my husband was going through.

Bald spots came and went, as did men. When I didn't have to wear full wigs, telling the men I went out with wasn't normally a problem. But after age forty, when I lost all my hair and had to start wearing wigs all the time, it was a fearsome issue – not just telling a date, but telling my friends, too.

I've Got a Secret

Most women who find they have alopecia areata try to hide it for as long as they can. Paula says: "I believe that most people don't want to know about my condition. It's too uncomfortable for them to imagine. So I had been trying to hide my condition from everyone for about a year, not even letting my husband know how bad it was (he finally saw when I came out of the shower and the bath towel I had wound around my head fell off). But then my two-year-old niece lost all her hair with alopecia universalis. I announced that I had it, too. Now my daughter has it and since I need to set an example for her, I am always upfront and ready to use the word 'alopecia.' "

Barbara, fifty-three, a CPA, shared her story through tears: "When my bald spots progressed to the point where I had to start wearing wigs, my husband told me he didn't find me attractive any longer and left me." I can't help but feel that the guy did her a favor by leaving. If he can't deal with this, what would happen if she ever became seriously ill and needed his care? What if she was in a disfiguring accident, had a stroke, or lost an arm or leg? Good riddance. Now she can find someone who cares about her for who she is, not what's on her head.

Susan, thirty-eight, a married mother of two, says she wishes her own mother didn't know, because she is very unsupportive. "Mom criticizes my wigs as if there is no reason I can't have the beautiful locks of my twenties. She asks me why I have this problem. I'm guessing she feels guilty and secretly thinks that somehow it's her fault – maybe she passed the 'bald gene' on to me. That's got to be very hard for her."

Nicole tells me that if someone asks her she will be truthful about her alopecia, but there are some people she will *never* tell about her worsening condition. "After I started wearing a wig, I actually moved from my home town in Colorado to another state because I was determined to avoid the classmates and friends who I grew up with and who knew me when I had thick, honey-blonde hair. I want them to think of me the way I was then, not the way I am now. So I didn't go to my ten-year high school reunion. I probably won't go to my twentieth, either. Yes, I have a great wig, but I'm afraid they will be able to tell. These kids were gossipy and always horribly delighted with others' misfortunes. Maybe they have grown into nicer people now, but I am feeling too vulnerable to expose myself to the possibility of being fodder for gossip and unkind remarks."

We have to face the fact that some people, including our husbands, close friends, and family, will not be able to deal with our alopecia. Sometimes it's because they're scared; they don't know how to handle it. Other times it's because they are more concerned about how you look than who you are inside. They're embarrassed to be seen with you or be your friend. They're not embarrassed for *you*, but for *themselves*. These people are superficial because they don't feel secure within themselves. They can't accept you as you are. Remember that losing a friend, boyfriend or husband like this not necessarily a bad thing. You want someone who is there for you through thick and thin – and bald.

How and When to Tell

You're dating a man and he affectionately reaches to arrange a strand of hair behind your ear, or to caress the nape of your neck. You flinch.

A coworker inspects you and says, "Wasn't your hair shorter yesterday?" You reply, "Um, it grows fast," as you try to remember which wig you had on then, and silently curse yourself for your lack of continuity.

Your dad says, "Hey, what's that on top of your head?" Your hand flies to your hair. Is it a bald spot, or a bug?

In the past, these were the only times I told people: when they were going to find out anyway. I'd start by saying something like, "I have something to tell you – I don't have hair anywhere." Quickly, before they get too panicky, I continue, "It's not catching. It's an autoimmune disorder...wait, where are you going?"

But now that I'm braver and more self-assured, I might tell someone just for the shock value. Like when they're complaining about getting a little thin on top, or if they're bemoaning a bad hair cut. It's kind of fun to see people's reactions.

One of my guy friends who was unaware of my condition was continually griping about the lack of hair atop his head. "Stop complaining," I said. "You have more hair than I do!" He looked at me and laughed. "No, really!" I said. " I have no hair anywhere!" After I explained, the size of his pupils went back to normal and he felt thankful for his sparse growth.

My girlfriends are so comfortable about my condition that they don't even think about it anymore – they cheerfully complain to me about hair triumphs and disasters on their own heads. However, sometimes I enjoy reminding them that I would gladly suffer their worst hair day if I could have mine back again!

Be courageous. It's one of the only places left uncrowded.

Dame Anita Roddic, Founder of The Body Shop

Natasha, twenty-six, a teacher, relates her experience telling her friend, Dee: "Even though I felt close to Dee as if she were my sister, I found it hard to tell her about my alopecia. I think it was because we were always having so much fun together, laughing, dancing and singing. I knew that if I told her about my hair, it would be a serious time and I would probably cry and feel sad. When I finally told Dee, her reaction was one of support and some hurt feelings that I hadn't told her before. This was my first true lesson in friendship; that sharing the tough times is equally as important as sharing the good times."

Becca, thirty, an insurance manager, told me that she had mixed reactions from friends, from shock and encouragement to bursting into tears. "My favorite reaction was from my good friend Yvonne who said with much relief, ' Is that all? Jeez, I thought it was a brain tumor!'"

Even if we're okay about our condition, it's hard to deal with the reactions of others, however well-meaning. "The times I have told a trusted friend have been very awkward," relates Paula. "I usually explain that my alopecia is under control and that my daughter and niece are the really the ones to sympathize with. I feel like a coward when I tell them this – I just can't deal with the grave sympathy that people offer."

The workplace can have its own set of horrors. Kathy talked about her experience with her co-workers: "After dealing with growing bald patches, I finally bit the bullet and got a wig. The first day I wore it, I cried all the way to work. As I walked from my car to my building, a girl from work fell in step with me, asking what was wrong. I was so choked up I couldn't talk, and just pointed to my head. She enthusiastically told me my new "hair" looked beautiful and natural. I felt a little better, but when I got off the elevator our receptionist looked at me funny and I started crying again. When I looked up several women were surrounding me, telling me how great the wig looked. I ran into my office, embarrassed to be the center of attention. Later, my boss stopped in and made positive comments about my hair, too. I wanted to tell them all to shut up! It went on all day. It was horrible. Now, six months later, the same people tell me they can't remember what I looked like before I had the wig, and no one fusses over me anymore. It's all okay now."

Then there are the people you don't even know. One night I was at a cocktail party when the elegant woman standing next to me said, "Is all that beautiful hair yours?" Although I thought this was somewhat rude, I replied sweetly, "Yes, it's mine, bought and paid for." Then I told her briefly about my condition. "Oh, I wish I had that!" she chirped. "Different hairdos, no blowdrying, no leg shaving!" I know she was trying to make me feel good and covering up her embarrassment, but to wish it on herself was a little extreme.

Kathy says, "I occasionally find that strangers stop me and compliment me on my hair and I am flummoxed every time, especially when stuck with them on an elevator at work. My boyfriend, Steve, gets mad at me for telling people it's a wig, but I have a hard time lying. He thinks I should just say thank you. So I tried that...about a month ago I was coming out of Costco and there was an older man that was bald on top, checking receipts at the exit. As I walked up to him, he enthusiastically said, "Boy, am I jealous!" "Of what?" I asked cautiously, thinking he was looking at something in my cart, which contained nothing particularly exciting. He said, "I'm jealous of all that thick, beautiful hair you have. I wish I had hair like that!" Steve would have been proud of me that time, because I just said, "Thank you," and left. Afterwards, I thought how I would have loved to tell him that I knew how he could get some of that exact same hair and we could be like twins!"

Barbara, a lovely sixty-two-year-old who travels extensively said, "I was at a beautiful hotel in France during the summer with some friends and it was ninety-five degrees. Everyone went out to the pool, and I was in a quandary. I knew I would get too hot with my wig on, but I didn't want anyone to see me with just a bandana or hat. Truth be told, I didn't especially want anyone to see me in a swimming suit, either! So I put on my wig, a hat, shorts and a top, and sat in the shade with my margarita so I wouldn't cook. It turns out I didn't have to worry about the way I looked. You should have seen some of the people who dared to wear swim suits. Ugh. It made me think that if I'd had *two* margaritas, I might have taken off my wig!"

There are a myriad other people you will probably want to tell: your chiropractor (if your hair isn't taped on securely, when he cracks your neck it may fly across the room);

your masseuse (I bring a soft turban in my purse to wear and switch to that before I get on the table. It always slips or comes off, but at least it's dark); the people at the bank (short hair one week, long the next...should you let them guess?), your eye doctor ("Did you know you don't have any eyelashes?" Is this a trick question?).

So, it's really up to you when you tell someone. There's no rule that says when, why or where. After all, hair loss is your own private business and not something you need to disclose right off the bat – or ever, if you don't feel like it!

"For me, it's a really big deal to tell someone about my hair, so I have to trust them implicitly," says Natasha. "It's not the sort of thing I can just drop into a conversation— 'The weather is nice today, and by the way, I wear a wig.' I have to hold them dear to my heart, and even then I have to wait until I've had two glasses of wine!

"I usually start by telling them something like this," continues Tash. 'You're a really good friend and I love you, which is why there is something I need to tell you. I want you to know the real me and I don't want to keep secrets from you and...' and then it all spills out. You'd think I was telling them I had seven days to live, with the amount of seriousness I give it!"

Separating the Men from the Boys

Maybe the most important support we receive (or don't receive) is from the men in our lives. Our fathers are the first males we look to, to help us feel good about being a girl – and all the accoutrements that go along with it. If they don't accept us without hair, how can we feel attractive to other men? Some girls who had alopecia at an early age were fortunate to have daddies that loved them no matter what.

Others are not as lucky.

Tash related this story: "I was twelve and had my first real crush on a fourteen-year-old boy. I thought he was so mature and handsome and I was certain I was in love with him. He knew I wore a wig, as his parents were friends with mine. This gave me the courage to ask him out since I wouldn't have to go through the ordeal of telling him. His answer was no. 'Why?' I asked. He told me it was because I wore a wig.

"Through sobs, I told my Dad why I was so upset. Dad 'consoled' me by saying,

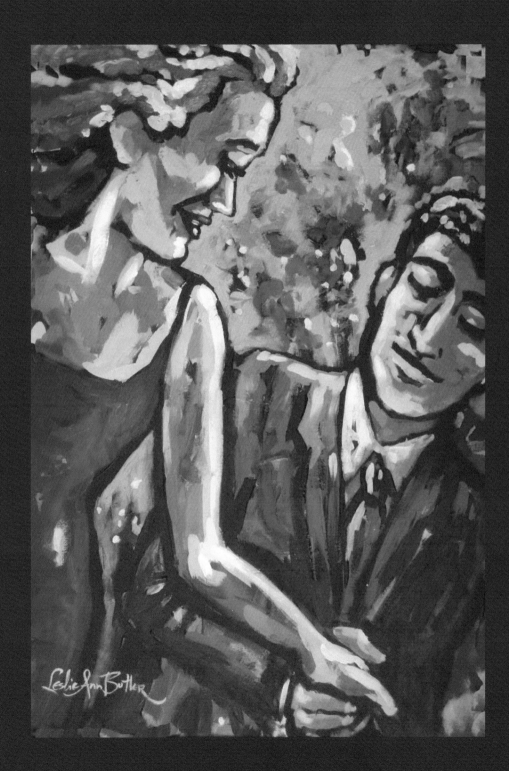

'Well, you wouldn't want to go out with him if *he* wore a wig, would you?' Only twelve years old, and the two men I loved most in the world had rejected me because I wore a wig."

I didn't have alopecia when I was little, but like so many of us, I have had to face the same gruesome fate: to tell any man who might get close to me about my condition.

I had dated Sean twice. As we chatted on the phone, he jokingly told me that I was so foxy that I would even look good bald. Hesitating only a few seconds, I decided this was the perfect lead-in. "Well, I *am* bald!" I blurted out. After what seemed like several hours of silence, I helpfully offered a bit more information as to how it all happened. Another long silence. He mumbled something like, " Er, my dog just threw up," and the line went dead. I never heard from him again. As I think back on that experience, I would have to say that it's probably better to tell someone face-to-face, and ideally to have developed some degree of mutual trust and understanding. Unfortunately, it doesn't guarantee that the guy will be any more receptive to your condition, and he might be very uncomfortable if he's trying to process this while figuring out how to make a speedy exit.

Mike, whom I had been seeing for a few weeks, took me to a hip new restaurant on the lake. He was lots of fun, and we always ate out because I don't really enjoy cooking, and he enjoyed declaring that he didn't know which side of the grater was the one that worked. Later that evening, as we began to cuddle in my foyer, he put his hand on my neck. I knew he would find the wig within moments, so I said, "I have something to tell you…" and explained the situation. I did my spiel about AA being an autoimmune disorder, and that it wasn't contagious or life threatening, but it left me without hair and I had to wear wigs. He snatched his hand away as if he had been burned, and his eyes were filled with shock and awe. Stuttering something like "I just…I must…I…I…well…you know…ah…gah…I am…bah…," he backed out the door with a deer-in-the-headlights look. Then he fell down the steps. (There were only three, so he didn't hurt himself too much.) He called four months later. I think the guilt was too much for him – he told me he had just found a cheese grater that worked on both sides, and thought I would get a kick out of that, ha ha. And after that, I never heard from him again.

Laura had a similar experience. "Paul and I had dated for three months and were getting really close. I had successfully kept his hands from going to the wrong places on my head or neck, but it was exhausting and nerve-wracking. We were lying on the bed, and I knew this was the time I had to tell him. I sat up and explained that I was wearing a wig and I had a condition that made my hair fall out. He was so sympathetic. He asked if I was sick, and I told him no, explaining about alopecia. Okay, good, I thought – he didn't burst out laughing or run away screaming. He was kind of quiet, and he got up, still acting very sweet. I was hoping he'd stay, but he walked out the door after giving me a (not passionate) kiss; I was hopeful that he would be okay about it. However, the next day he didn't call. Or the next, or the next. I finally realized I had been dumped."

Rohnn (pronounced Ron) was an extremely proper (or as my friends like to say, uptight) man. We had dated for almost a year, when he finally declared it was time for him to go on to more hirsute pastures. "I don't feel very good about myself for saying this," he said, "but I just can't deal with your lack of hair." I was shocked. I had been having so much fun with my wig wardrobe – short, long, in-between, gold, black, red, strawberry blonde, platinum – that I imagined he was getting a kick out of it, too. It turns out that Rohnn was terrified and confused, not knowing what color, style and length of hair he would find upon my head from one day to the next, and the strain was just too much for him. (Now that hair extensions are the new trend, there are a *lot* of women confusing people with their hairdos! Just look at People Magazine and you'll see the same face with a number of different styles and colors!) Anyway, self-admittedly shallow Rohnn found a hairy woman several years ago. I hadn't seen him until the other night at a dressy party where I had on one of my luscious long blonde wigs, the beauty of which my wig and styling provider extraordinaire, Brenda Kay, was responsible for. He approached me and drew me toward him. "LeslieAnn! How lovely to see you!" he cried. As he pulled me closer for an air kiss, he whispered, "I see that your hair has grown back. It's beautiful!" Ah! Having a beautiful hair system (thank you BK!) is the best revenge!

Fortunately, I've found that with men, negative reactions are the exception rather

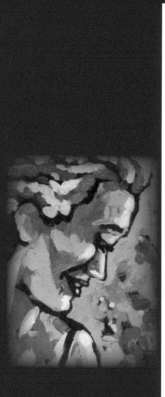

than the rule. After I screw up my courage, my experiences telling men have been very positive. One handsome Lake Oswego man was entranced when I told him. "Oooo! *Seck-zee!*" he enthused. Nervously I backed away, certain he was eager to check out this alopecia universalis, universally. Another man thought it was wonderful that I wore many different colors and styles of wigs. " Woo hoo," he told me, "It's my own harem!"

Then there's the guy who presents you with calm acceptance. I think that's the best kind of reception. He appreciates your openness. He is quick to say that it doesn't matter, and means it.

Most of the women I spoke to had good things to say about their partners and husbands, like Kathy: "When I told my boyfriend about my first spot, he immediately started teasing me. But when he realized how much that hurt me, he made a one-eighty. Now he constantly tells me it doesn't matter to him whether or not I have hair, that he will love me if I go completely bald. He lets me cry on his shoulder when I need to."

Amber Humphrey, who sells hair systems and has alopecia herself, told her husband (the most attractive bachelor in town) almost as soon as she met him. "A woman's attitude makes all the difference. I know I'm a gift from God, and let him know it, too!" Fifteen years later she says their marriage still feels like a honeymoon.

Nicole says her husband is great. "He makes me feel beautiful. He is the only person I am totally comfortable with bare headed. He offered to shave his head for me. I told him it was okay, and I really appreciated the offer – but he doesn't have that much hair in the first place! Sometimes I think of us sitting on the couch together, a couple of baldies, and how that is kind of cute."

One woman decided to tell her new guy via email. I am a big fan of email, and think this might be a good way to do it. You can explain what alopecia areata is, your personal history, and how you deal with it, and how hard it is to have to tell people. This gives him time to read what you say, digest it, even do his own research if he sincerely wants to understand your condition.

Remember that when you first tell your guy, it will be a bit of a shock. A common reaction to such news is to pull away at first. A bit of apprehension is normal. Give him some time to process the information.

And if you get dumped? Join the club. You don't have to be physically perfect to have a happy relationship. There are a lot of beautiful, perfect-appearing women out there who get dumped or deserted for no apparent reason. It happens to everyone, hair or not. But if you get rejected because of alopecia areata, who wants the guy anyway? You're better off without fair-weather boyfriends.

You younger women and teenage girls may believe that you will never meet a man who will accept you, let alone love you, with alopecia. I'm telling you right now, your odds of meeting someone who will fall head over heels in love with you, with or without hair, are very high! Stay open, and don't obsess about it. The less your condition bothers you, the less it will bother others. Many, *many* women meet and marry attractive, quality men *after* their hair loss.

What if you want to keep your AA a secret? You could try it, but I don't know how long you can get away with it. There will come a time when your sweetie will want to run hands through your hair, or take a shower with you, or give you a head rub. You could grab his hand and guide it to your rosy, dimpled knee, but that will look pretty suspicious after you've done it a couple of times. At that point, hopefully he knows you well enough to think he's a pretty lucky guy for being with you, and wants to continue the relationship. Keeping secrets is a burden and not such a good way to enter into a potentially promising relationship. Go ahead, and tell him in your own sweet way. He might have a little secret for you, too.

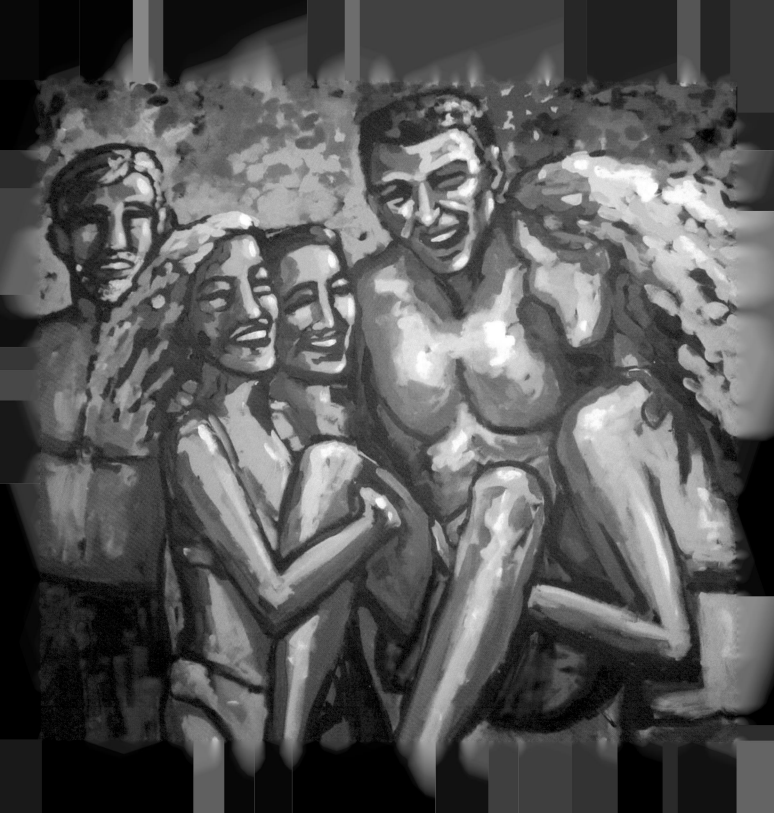

CHAPTER SEVEN

Separation Anxiety

If you don your wig every morning with your underwear like I do, it's scary to think about the possibility of losing it in front of someone – be it friend or stranger. It can happen. Mine came off when an ex-boyfriend got mad at me and jerked my hair. Guess he forgot it wasn't attached. Instead of causing me pain, it came off in his hands. While he stood there not knowing what to do next, I ran. That's one reason he's an ex.

Here are a few examples of what other people have experienced:

"I was mowing the lawn and caught my wig on a low-hanging tree branch. It pulled my hair off and startled, I let go of the lawnmower which continued to move at a brisk clip toward the sidewalk and a passing pedestrian. I stood there frozen, not knowing whether to grab my wig from the tree branch or go after the lawnmower! The guy walking by was nice enough to rescue the mower while I fumbled with replacing my hair." —*Julie, forty-four, advertising executive*

"I was in the car with a date – we hadn't been seeing each other for very long and he didn't know I wore a wig. We had to stop suddenly in traffic, and the car behind us crashed into us. Neither of us was hurt, but at the moment of impact my wig flew off and into my lap. My boyfriend looked over to see if I was okay, and saw the wig. He yelled, "Oh my God, it's a rat!" And jumped out of the car. I hurriedly threw my wig back on and sat there, laughing." — *Janice, twenty-four, dog groomer*

" It was a really windy day and a giant gust of wind caught my wig just right – I guess I didn't tape it down well enough. It flew off my head and sailed into the busy street. Cars were swerving to miss it! Instinctively, I threw my coat over my head and stood there, waiting for my wig to cross the street so I could go after it without being hit. A jogger rescued it and returned it to me. I was so mortified. I put it under my coat and made tracks out of there." — *Maddy, seventeen, student*

"I was in the library in the shelves, looking for some books to take on a trip. I had on new flip flops and somehow they caught on the carpet. Suddenly, I crashed into the shelf, knocking my wig off my head. Lightning fast I crouched down to hide as I grabbed my hair off the floor and shoved it back on my head. Then I slowly rose and carefully looked around to see if anyone noticed. There were two people who I'm sure heard the crash and looked, but discreetly were now engaged in conversation, ignoring me. Yes, I was embarrassed, but I pretended like nothing happened, retrieved my books and my dignity, and walked out. When I got to the car I found out I had put my wig on crooked so that one side was about four inches shorter than the other!" — *Angela, thirty-two, travel consultant*

"The only time my wig has ever slipped was when I took a self-defense class. As I was learning how to throw off an attacker who had me pinned to the ground, my wig slipped sideways. Someone said, 'Oh, her hair!' I turned red and fixed it right away, but then everyone knew it was a wig. Fortunately, no one acted like it was unusual and it was okay." — *Nicole, thirty-eight, sales*

"I did something really dumb. I can't believe I did this! Before I went into the gym at my club to work out, I pulled my wig back into a low pony tail to keep the hair out of my face. After my workout, I was walking out of the weight room and wanted to let my hair down, so I pulled out the elastic band. Unconsciously, I tugged on it hard, just as if I was pulling on my own growing hair (I was newly wearing wigs), and tore the wig right off my head! I dashed into a conveniently-located ladies' room!" — *Angie, twenty-two, customer service rep*

A moving or flying wig can happen to anyone, but thankfully there are ways to keep it to a minimum or prevent it all together. Tapes come in varying strengths, and liquid bonding adhesives can really hold a hair system to your scalp, even if you sweat. And you can count on real security with a vacuum-based wig. It will stay on until you take it off. Non-vacuum silicone-based wigs are usually pretty secure if they have been carefully custom fit to your head.

Sex and Other Sports

I have had nightmares about making love sans wig, waking up very relieved it was only a dream. Maybe there's something wrong with me, or maybe it's just plain vanity, but I feel sexier with hair on my head.

Yes, sometimes it comes loose. One time after I got up, I looked in the mirror to find that my wig was on sideways. That tape just didn't hold firmly enough! However, I am certain that my man was too distracted with other parts of me to even notice.

Samantha, a twenty-eight-year-old executive, says, "When my husband wants to get intimate, I wear my wig. Otherwise I just don't feel sexy. I try to keep it on while we're making love, but it moves around – so instead of enjoying myself, I worry about it falling off. He says it's okay...but it's just *not* okay for me. He says, you take everything else off – just take the hair off, too!"

Judy, a thirty-eight-year-old banker, doesn't wear her wig at those intimate times.. "There's no way I can have sex without my wig coming off! Worrying about it made me inhibited. So now, I just don't wear it. My boyfriend is totally accepting of that."

"I don't wear anything on my head while making love or sleeping," Kathy says. "If Steve hadn't been with me through it from the beginning, it might be a different story."

Nicole says, "I have never worn a wig during sex. In fact, before I lost my hair, it was so fine that it sometimes caused problems. It would go up my husband's nose, and believe me, *that* was not sexy! It was probably a relief for him not to have to mess with it."

Donna, fifty-two, a receptionist, told me, "If the person you're making love with can't deal with your bald head, that's his problem, not yours! But don't be surprised if your partner accepts your bald head – he might even find it sexy!"

There's one thing about baldness, it's neat.

Don Herold, Cartoonist

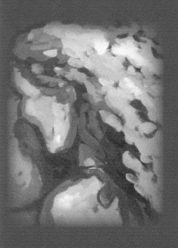

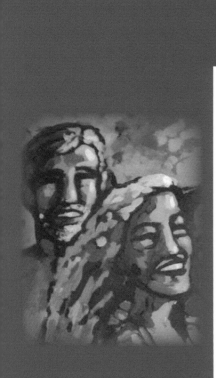

In her experience, Hannah has found that men don't tend to notice those things, or even care about them at all. "My boyfriend is a wonderful person and I feel completely comfortable with him. I can look him in the eye and have him touch my head."

As for other sports, I don't play soccer, tennis, swim, or bungee jump or juggle chainsaws while hanging from an airplane – but when I know I'm going to be sweating (like hiking, lifting weights or bicycling), I like to wear either a synthetic or human hair wig with wefting or netting because the silicone-based wigs are too hot for me. The synthetics are easy to wash and wear.

Kathy used to be quite active before she started wearing a wig. "It's uncomfortable. It's like a hairy hat. And it's hot. I bought an inexpensive synthetic wig to wear to the gym, but sadly, I have never gone because I know it would be so uncomfortable. I hate it when I'm outdoors on a warm day and sweat is dripping from underneath my wig. I think it would be lots worse if I were at the gym *trying* to sweat!"

I understand Kathy's concerns. However, most gyms are equipped with fans and air conditioning, and copious amounts of perspiration may not be a problem. Don't forget, you can duck into a stall in the bathroom, pull off your wig, towel off your scalp, then plop it on again. It works!

For people whose concerns include participating in very active sports like tennis, soccer and swimming, vacuum or suction wigs will stay secure in most conditions. Heavy-duty tapes and adhesives will do the trick, too. "I am pretty active, so I wear strong tapes and adhesives. There is no way my hair is coming off," says Amber. "In fact, it stays on for up to four weeks. I treat it just like natural hair, wash and wear."

Whatever you do, don't let your wig get in the way of doing the things you love. We all have to adapt, and then be thankful for our health and the wonderful options that are available to us today. Choose to celebrate, live and love your life. If Miss Molly can do it, so can you!

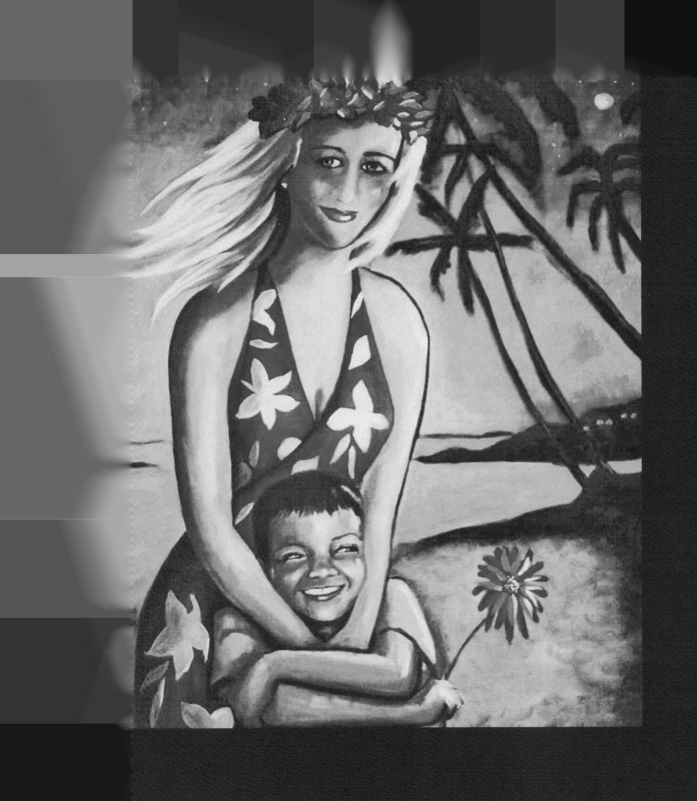

CHAPTER EIGHT

Baby Blues

Having a child with alopecia may be more difficult than having it yourself. You feel helpless. You can't kiss it and make it better. And worse, you may blame yourself because of the possible hereditary factors, even though odds are against that. The National Alopecia Areata Foundation says that there is more than an 90% chance you will *not* pass alopecia on to your child.

"At first, I was overwhelmed with anxiety," says Mimi, twenty-nine, a restaurant hostess with a four-year-old daughter who had just developed alopecia areata. "Was this *my* fault? Will it go away? How will this affect her later, in grade school, high school? This loss of her hair can interfere with the development of her identity. She is sometimes mistaken for a little boy. Other kids can be so cruel. I went through the whole thing with trying to find a cure. The injections, the creams. It was so hard for her, I gave up. I could see that the doctors didn't have a clue as to what to do for her."

Paula said just when she felt she had come to terms with her own alopecia, her six-year-old daughter, Angela, developed it. "That was a dirty deal," she said. "I feel so guilty because obviously, I passed on the gene to her. She didn't notice her own spots – I found them while brushing her hair. I had thought about this conversation a million times and knew how to approach her. 'Honey, you know I have alopecia and your cousin has it too…

it runs in our family. Also, you know how much we are alike? Well, I've noticed you have some spots like I do.' I was expecting shock and tears, but she was soooo underwhelmed! 'I don't care, I can't even see the spots,' she said. We started our own grooming routine – she would cover my spots with a sponge brush and makeup paint, and then I would do hers. I just hope that her healthy attitude carries into her teens." If things get worse, Paula says, they will look for wigs together. "I will casually say something like, 'Someday I may have a wig and I'll get something really fun – maybe go blonde! Will you come with me?'"

Liz's daughter is just coming into her teen years. A very difficult time for any young woman, add alopecia areata and it can be quite a challenge. "Autoimmune diseases run in our family, and Emily not only has alopecia, but arthritis," says Liz, forty-four. "I feel terribly guilty that she has to deal with this; I think she has more than enough on her plate. I realize alopecia is not physically painful, but emotional pain can be even worse. Moms are supposed to be able to kiss their kids and make everything better. I can't do that with alopecia."

It would be great if all kids had the healthy attitude toward their own AA as Janet's sixteen-year-old daughter, Caroline, who has coped with it for three years. She tells people about alopecia this way: "Some people have lots of zits, some people have crossed eyes, some people have super hairy legs. For me, I have bald patches. I lose my hair in clumps. It doesn't hurt, and it doesn't change who I am."

Kids and Teasing

Because kids are the way they are, it's best to prepare your child right away for the possibility of being teased. Remind her that children will always find something to tease about, whether it's her name, glasses, a pimple, her height. The best thing to do is ignore it. I know that sounds simplistic, but when the bully doesn't get the satisfaction of seeing her cry, get angry, or at least become uncomfortable, there's no reward. Here's a story from someone who wants to remain anonymous:

"My daughter Ellen, who has alopecia, used to ride the bus to a private school in New York. One day on the school bus, a rich kid with a famous father called her 'baldy.'

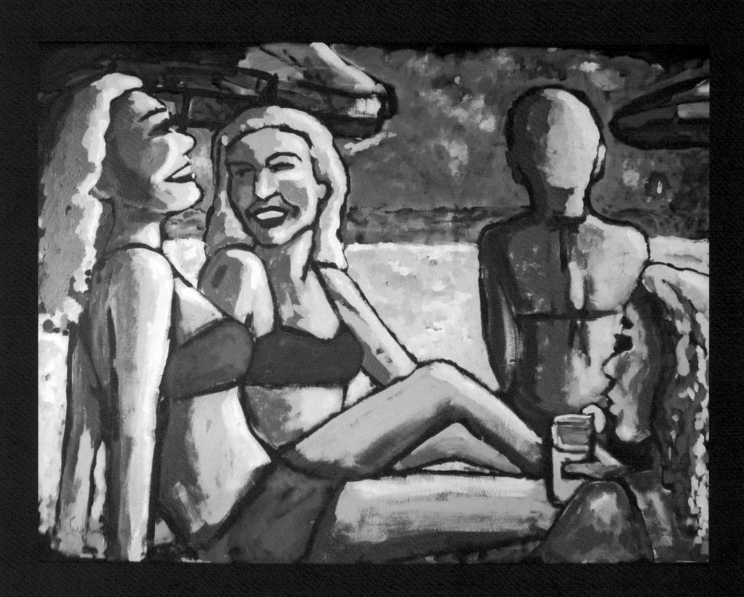

She had been prepared and was ready – we taught her that if it doesn't push your buttons, it won't be any fun for the teaser. So no matter how much it hurts, or how embarrassed you are, ignore it. So she completely ignored "Rich and Famous Jr.," even though he continued to tease her. The other kids on the bus were silent. Finally one boy said, 'Hey, guy, knock it off.' He did, and the incident passed. About four months later, when Jr.'s father, ex-wife and current girlfriend were getting a lot of negative press, someone on the bus started teasing him about the women in his dad's life. Everyone was shocked when Ellen stood up and said, 'Boy, if you can't find something better to tease a guy about than his mother, you are really pathetic.' From then on, these kids had enormous respect for Ellen. If anyone gave her a hard time about her lack of hair they were ostracized."

Generally, when other people understand the condition, it takes all the scariness and mystery out of it and becomes 'normal.' Liz says that her daughter's classmates have never teased her. "They've actually been quite kind and expressed concern for her. This may be because Emily has been with the same group for the past four years, in a program for gifted children. I'm concerned about the change next year – Emily will enter seventh grade and will be with many kids who know nothing about her condition."

In this case my advice would be to teach the school, starting with the nurse. Don't talk to the children directly because it separates your daughter from her peers. One idea is to approach the school with the possibility of a succinct but informative mailing to the parents so they can privately educate their children.

"I think if my teachers had known and made an effort to work with my parents, my life at junior high and high school would have been a lot easier," Susan, twenty-four, a management trainee says. " I didn't let AA stop me from doing what I wanted to do – I was a cheerleader and in theater – but people were always watching with morbid fascination to see if somehow my wig would come off. Fortunately, it never happened during a game. But it happened other times. I think if a kid is brave enough, she should make an informational video, or write a speech and give it to her classmates, and that would head off problems. Most kids are just curious and once they know what's happening and can ask questions in a positive environment, they'll accept it."

I highly recommend a visual aid from NAAF: a seven-minute video called "This Weird Thing That Makes My Hair Fall Out – Alopecia Areata." It's available free to any children who need a way to share their feelings about AA with friends, family, peers, schoolmates, principals and teachers. Ask them to send one of their brochures for children as well.

Belinda, a teen, has alopecia universalis and tells me that she started losing her hair when she was nine. "It took me about five years to come to terms with it," she says. "For girls, it's one of the top ten worst things that could possibly happen. But you know what? It isn't number one! I decided it wasn't the end of the world. I wore wigs for a while, but they were hot and itchy. Now, I go to school football games and dances without a wig, scarf or hat. Sure, I get my share of stares, but deep down inside I know that I am just as pretty as any other girl on the dance floor. Nothing will change that."

Hannah's experience with classmates wasn't as positive as Susan's or Emily's. "I have always had alopecia areata and still live with it, but from age nine to age thirteen, I had totalis: no hair on my head, no eyebrows and no eyelashes. Children and teenagers, especially girls, can be very cruel. When I was in elementary and middle school, they would say things like, 'Did you know you don't have any eyebrows?' A lot of people assumed I had cancer because I wore wigs, and I always wondered how they could be so rude to someone they thought had cancer!" She says, "I developed a stronger sense of self early on than most kids, because I knew that I was not defined by my outward appearance. That doesn't mean I don't deal with vanity issues every day, though!"

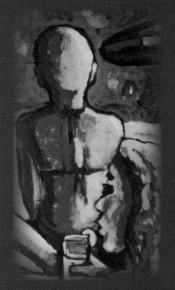

How to Help

If your child wants to wear a wig, get her at least one quality hairpiece as soon as you can, and have it styled to look natural. Many hairpieces are too thick and full – this is especially obvious on little heads.

"Emily has patchy bald spots – her alopecia hasn't progressed to the point where she has to wear wigs. Her main concern is finding hairstyles that camouflage the spots," says Liz. "We're making sure the school knows she has my permission to wear hats if she needs to. The choice of wearing a hat, wig, or nothing at all, is Emily's. She's the one who needs

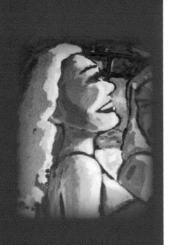

to feel in control. I think the emotional aspects of being a teenage girl with hair loss may be the most difficult thing she's ever going to face."

I suggested to Liz and Emily that since she'll be going to a new school with a group of new kids, it might be better to put Emily into a nice wig now before she meets them. If she waits and things get worse, she will have the difficulty of explaining the change to the other children. There is also the option of hair extensions which can cover the spots.

Paula talks about her girls and vanity issues: "My daughters' cousin who is in grade school taught them that hair or no hair, people are the same. 'I don't care if she wears her wig or not,' one of my daughters said, 'she's fun either way!' They all play dress-up and makeup – but I think they know that's just the outside, and what's important is on the inside."

Hannah advises adolescent girls to get involved with a support group. "When I was younger, I didn't want to get involved with NAAF or go to support group meetings because I didn't want to acknowledge that I was different from my friends. I think this was a mistake, and if I had it to do over I would meet others who are in my same situation. It's always wonderful to have friends who really understand you.

"I would also tell other girls it's important to remember that alopecia doesn't have to define you, and that it's okay to want to cover it up. It's not vanity – it's just wanting to blend in, and that's okay. It's also okay to let yourself get angry and feel like what's happening to you isn't fair. And if it's really hard, it's okay to go to therapy. I did, and I recommend it."

All in all, the best thing to do for your daughter (or son) is to help her develop a strong self-image. When she knows she is intelligent, talented and special she will not blame herself for being different. With your help and guidance she will accept that she is different, but for the better.

And, as Liz says, "We need to allow our children to be actively involved in the decision-making that goes along with having alopecia areata. How involved depends on her age and maturity, but she absolutely must be involved. How we parents feel isn't nearly as important as how the child feels."

Paula has told her daughter that everyone has *something*. "It's the human condition. If you have alopecia, you're lucky in some ways because you know what it is that you must deal with – and otherwise you're perfectly healthy. In fact, alopecia means your body is working *overtime* to keep you healthy!" She also likes to tell Angela that because of her alopecia, she is developing a sympathetic outlook. "You will always have more sympathy and understanding for people who have disabilities or other factors that make them feel or look different. Alopecia teaches us to look beyond and beneath the surface."

Hannah agrees. "I had to grow up quickly and in a lot of ways. I think I am a more empathetic person than a lot of other people my age. Having had this intense life experience so young definitely increases your understanding of the world around you."

Finding Children's Wigs

Hannah's advice is clear, "Do *not* go to just *any* wig store, because in my experience they don't specifically deal with hair loss due to alopecia or chemotherapy and they can be very insensitive. Always go to someone who specializes in hair loss disorders. It's worth the money to get a custom-fitted wig, especially for children who are active. I was able to swim and go to ballet classes with mine."

There are a few places that create wigs especially for children; the Resource section has contact information. For financially disadvantaged children eighteen years and younger who have long-term hair loss, you may find help from these two non-profit organizations: Locks of Love, and Wigs for Kids; and for children and teens in Oregon, the Angel Hair Foundation.

Where is Mom's Hair?

How do you handle it with the kids when you have alopecia areata? If small children and babies are used to seeing you with hair, they can become fearful when your hair changes or falls out. The opposite is true, too – if your little one is used to seeing you with patchy spots or completely bald and you show up with a wig, this can cause uncertainty.

One woman who had a baby who didn't recognize her when she wore a wig solved this dilemma by developing little rituals that would help her child recognize her no matter what. For example, she used special pet names, songs and little rhymes that no one else

Better a bald head than no head at all.

Seamus MacManus, Author

would say. She let her baby play with her wigs and hats, letting him touch them and put them on teddy bears. He was never afraid again, no matter which wig she wore!

Julie says that one day her three-year-old niece walked in on her while putting on makeup – and she hadn't put on her wig yet. "Anna stood there without saying anything, and I was not sure what to do. When I hesitatingly said, 'I look different, don't I?' Anna replied, 'You look beautiful.' She was so sincere, I got tears in my eyes."

Julie continues, "My four-year-old son, however, is a different story. He doesn't like it when I don't have my wig on. He insists I put it on right away. 'You look better with it on!' He says. I guess I have to agree with him!"

For older children, openness is generally the best option. Marlene, a forty-one-year-old mother, told this story: "One day when I was picking my twelve-year-old son up from school, one of his classmates asked, 'Is it true you don't have hair?' 'Yes,' I said, and I took off my wig. I smiled, explaining briefly about alopecia. The boy who asked simply said, 'OK.' Later I asked my son if I had embarrassed him, and he said, 'No, I'm glad you did, because they were asking me and I didn't know what to say.'"

Some kids aren't so easy-going about their mom's AA. "My fourteen-year-old boy is extremely embarrassed if I go out of the house with a scarf or turban instead of my wig," says Mary Ann, a store manager. "It's funny, my fifteen-year-old daughter, who is obsessed with looks, doesn't care at all. But my son has made me promise to wear my wig if I go outside – especially in his environment, like school or clubs."

Dr. Manuel Casanova, Gottfried and Gisela Kolb Endowed Chair in Psychiatry and Associate Chair for Research at the Department of Psychiatry at the University of Louisville, has a teenage daughter with alopecia areata. He suggests that this is a perfect opportunity to teach the kids the mature way to deal with life's problems. "Don't get angry when your child complains and is embarrassed about your condition. Tell them that you don't need an excuse for your baldness. You are not ashamed, and you don't have to deny it. It's just a problem with your hair; people like you for *who you are*, not for your hair. Tell him or her that you understand how it feels to be embarrassed. Also tell him that if anyone notices, has questions, or teases him, to come and tell you. You will gladly answer their questions. Just remember that while outward appearances are sometimes

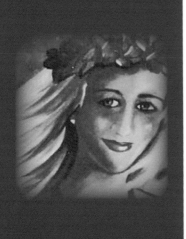

extremely important to teens and pre-teens, the real essence of being their parent goes far beyond what is visible. The lessons and guidance you provide, the examples of compromise and cooperation, and the focus on the intangible values are what they will look back on and draw from as they mature. Remember that they are children, as yet immature, and they're striving to define their own values, outlooks, and yes, prejudices. They look primarily to us as models to copy the parts they are comfortable with, and continually make choices (sometimes defying any logic or explanation!)."

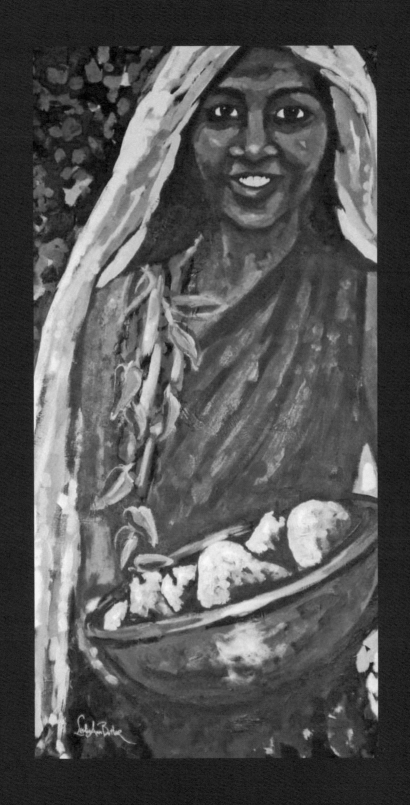

CHAPTER NINE

The Great Cover Up

Should you cover up, or not?

A lot of women with alopecia feel perfectly okay about going without hair or a hat, showing their bald heads to the world. This is great, and you have my complete support. On the other hand, if you don't want to show anyone how you look without hair, that's fine, too. A lot of women I've spoken to about the issue think there's something wrong with them if they don't feel comfortable letting it all hang out. I'm telling you right now, there isn't. We all have our comfort levels. For me, the number of people I will let see my bald head is about four that I can think of right now, including my doctor.

If you have enough patches that a windy day strikes fear in your heart, it's probably time to start wearing a wig, or maybe hair extensions will work for you. I remember how hard it was figuring out ways to camouflage my spots and avoiding situations like fast carnival rides, sticking your head out of a rapidly moving vehicle, or fast walking. "I have a really hard time covering my bald spots," admits Paula. "At my kids' soccer practice this fall, I didn't want to stand out in the wind to chitchat with other parents. I didn't happen to have a hat with me that day to cover up. Frankly, I feel funny always having to wear them.

"When I had to start wearing a wig, I just decided to think of it like brushing my teeth; putting it on every morning became a part of my daily routine. I didn't want to go out without it in public, and I don't think I'm less of a person for feeling that way," says Paula.

Kathy doesn't wear her wig at home. When she puts it on her dog knows she's going somewhere! When she first got her new hair, she placed it on a stand in her closet. Her dog saw it and figured it was another animal. She had to laugh when he barked at it hysterically for fifteen minutes until she put it back on her head and let him sniff it.

Some women use headbands, scarves and hats to cover patches and feel fine about always wearing them, making it part of their style. Long scarves and turbans can be quite exotic. There are also wigs made especially for women who can use their own hair, which I'll discuss later in this chapter.

The point is, do what you like and try to have fun with it!

Different Kinds of Wigs

Fortunately, hair system technology has come a long way since the late 1960's, a time when wigs and falls were very popular. Now you can get just about anything your budget will allow, from good-looking synthetics to custom-made European hair wigs. I have at least one of each, because they each have their place.

Synthetic

Synthetics are a definite requirement in my wig wardrobe. They're great for travel: shampoo them and they'll dry overnight, and you don't need to haul around curling irons and blowdriers. And I use them when I work out, because they're wash and wear. I've found that with daily wear they need to be washed at least once every two weeks. More if you're doing sweaty or dirty tasks.

The first thing to know about synthetic wigs is that they are great for short hairstyles – that is, above the collar – and not so great for longer styles. This is because synthetics are friction and heat sensitive, and they will frizz up from rubbing against your collar, neck or shoulders. You also have to be careful about opening oven doors, being anywhere near curling irons, and sunbathing in really hot weather. One woman

You could be one of those fabulous bald women who are all about the earrings.

Carrie Bradshaw,
Sex and the City

found out the hard way that the place to store her synthetic wig was not under the sink next to the hot water pipe! As Kathy says, "Stay away from the oven! And the barbecue too. Which is really inconvenient when you want to have guests over for dinner!"

A candlelight dinner may be romantic, but while you lean across the table to stare into your beloved's eyes, keep one eye on the candle! Waiting for our meal at a little bistro, I put my paper napkin down on the table and leaned toward my husband. Suddenly, I saw flames as first the napkin, and then my hair, caught on fire. There was gasping and shrieking throughout the dining room. And that was just me. Other diners watched in horrified delight at possibly their best dinner show ever. My husband picked up a full glass of ice water to throw on me as I was contemplating doing a drop and roll. Fortunately I got the fire out by smothering it with my jacket. I was unhurt, except for my ego. The wig, however, was trashed. Did I have another wig with me? Of course not; I had to walk around with a serious case of frizzies for another three days! That taught me to always bring a backup.

Another difficulty with many synthetics, especially light blonde tones, is shininess. They don't look natural in some kinds of light, especially in photographs taken with a flash. I've found that powdering them lightly will cut down the glare. I use regular face powder and stroke the puff over the top layer of hair. Darker colors are usually not a problem, but if you need to tame the shine on a dark wig, match the color with a matte powder eyeshadow and that will do the trick.

Contrary to popular belief, if you take good care of a short synthetic it will last you many months, perhaps even years. I have two that are a couple of years old and still look good. By the way, if you do happen to get fried frizzies, some experienced wig stylists can straighten them out for you.

Although synthetic wigs can last a long time with proper care, they often change color slightly. Sometimes blonde wigs can take on a pink cast. You can then use them for Halloween – or you can try treating them with Roux Fanciful rinse in shade or two darker than your wig. Roux Fanciful can be found at most large pharmacies (Walgreen's, for example) and beauty supply stores. It is very gentle and washes out each time you shampoo.

George Costanza: You fixed me up with a bald woman!

Elaine: Do you see the irony here? You're rejecting somebody because they're bald!

George: So?

Elaine: YOU'RE bald!

Seinfeld Episode: The Beard

Amy Gibson, head of Crown and Glory Enterprises, also handles synthetic wigs, including a line of wigs (Amy's Presence Coral Collection) that uses a product called CyberHair which claims to have the look and feel of human hair with the ease of styling of synthetic without the same "frizz factor" as Kanekalon or other synthetic hair. (But will it catch on fire?)

Synthetics can be machine made or hand-tied. The more hand tying in a wig, the more comfortable and lighter it will be – and more expensive. Both types are generally available at wig shops. You can also find some inexpensive synthetic wigs (some as low as $39) from catalogs and through the Internet. Beauty Trends and Paula Young are two companies I have ordered from, and been happy with. They have a variety of different styles, including the latest trendy ones. You'll find more in the Resources section of this book.

I recommend a monofilament top. It lets you make a part wherever you want, and looks like hair is growing out of your scalp. For a good synthetic wig with a mono top, you might have to pay about $250 and up. Sometimes you'll find the same wig at a discount or on sale if you check around. My favorite mono top synthetic wigs are by Rene of Paris, their Amore line, the Designer Series. There are also wigs that come with just a narrow strip of monofilament so you have the benefit of natural-looking hair growth, but the top can't be parted anywhere else. If you don't mind, you'll save a few dollars.

Human Hair

For hair styles that are collar length or longer, or those that require movement, your most natural look will be with a human hair wig. There are two kinds: pre-manufactured, and custom.

Pre-manufactured wigs are made from Asian and Indian hair. Of the two kinds, Indian is softer and easier to style, and depending on the color, can be virgin or processed hair. Asian hair is generally heavily processed and dyed. One of the advantages of pre-made wigs is availability – if a wig store has your color in stock, you can get it right away. Ordering one in your color will generally take only a few days. Get the closest

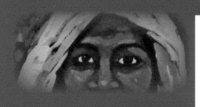

match to the color you want, because although these are human hair, recoloring them isn't that easy. Going darker isn't usually a problem, but going lighter is. I have been able to get some blonde streaks in this kind of wig by carefully applying L'Oreal hair color remover, but it's not as natural-looking as I would like.

Custom wigs are made to fit your head exactly, and the color is hand-picked. These wigs can be made with Asian, Indian or European hair. The most luxurious is European hair which is virgin, or unprocessed hair. Custom wigs will be considerably more expensive, and it will be about two to three months before you can put it on your head. This virgin hair can be easily colored with streaks, highlights or low lights.

I have both pre-made and custom wigs, and I have to say that because I am a blonde and generally wear my hair long, I like the custom ones best. However, I went for many years without a custom wig and got along just fine – so do what suits you and your budget. (Your insurance may cover the cost of your wig. To find out more about this, contact NAAF.)

Sizing

To find out your size, measure your head from your hairline (or where it would be) to above the nape of your neck, just below the occipital bone. Most ready-made wigs come in an "average" size, which is around 21.5 – 22.5". Small sizes are 21" and under, and large is over 22.5". My head falls in the "small" category. That means if I don't want my wig to bunch up in the back or poof out on top which happens with the Velcro sizing tabs, I might have to resize the premade wigs I buy. Wefted wigs (sown in rows), are easy to resize if you're at all handy with a needle. Simply remove one or two rows of wefting. Turn the wig inside out and using a pair of scissors, cut the elastic band close to the nape above and below the wefts you will remove. Cut the wefts from the elastic bands and then reattach the bands.

If you have a completely hand-tied wig, you should leave the resizing to your stylist. And of course, a custom-made wig is just that – designed to fit your head perfectly.

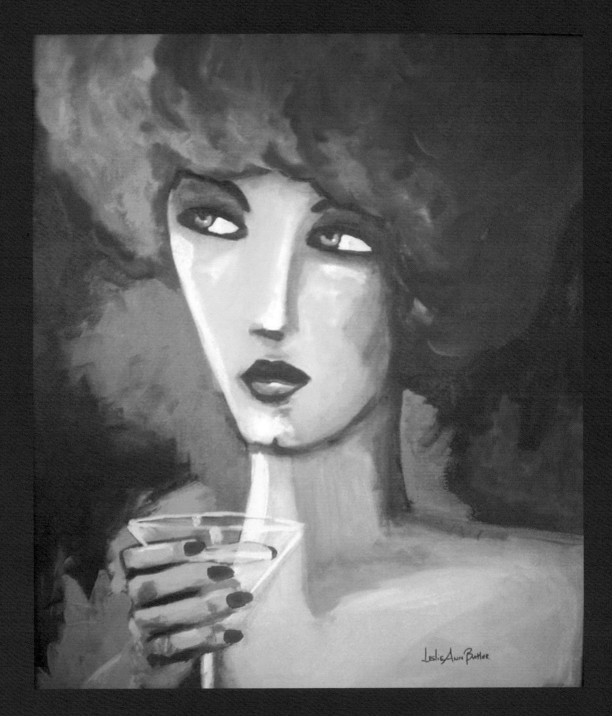

Color

If you buy your wig from a catalog or online, don't trust the colors you see in the pictures! Some companies will send you free color samples, and some have color rings you can purchase or borrow. You can also send a sample of your own hair, or hair from a wig that you like. One woman who had no hair sent a sample of her best friend's hair and now they have the same do's!

Types of Caps

Wefted

A few years ago, all wigs were wefted – that is, several strands of hair gathered at the top and sewn onto bands. This meant limited styling opportunities (the hair was sown in one direction only), and presented a problem for women who had no hair at all because scalp can show through the bands of wefting on a windy day. You can still purchase wefted wigs, and if you have some hair, this type kind can save you money. But be warned that they are not generally as natural-looking as hand-tied wigs. The best thing about wefted wigs is that the bands create "vents" and therefore, your head stays relatively cool on warm days. They can also be very lightweight.

Skin Top

This is wefted all over except the crown, which contains hair (usually synthetic) tied to mesh and covered with latex, giving the appearance of hair growing from scalp. Your real scalp doesn't show. I have found that it tends to look boxy and it's not easy to get a natural style from a skin top wig.

Monofilament Top

Individual hairs are hand-tied into fine, flesh-colored mesh. The color of your scalp shows through and generally looks quite natural.

Lace Front

I love my silicone base wig with its lace front! I can wear my hair pulled off my face and it looks like hair is growing out of my hairline. It's a little more fragile than wigs with regular reinforced front, but the lace strip can be repaired or replaced.

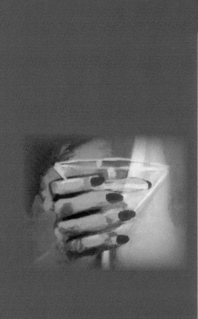

Molded Base

This is a soft, thin base that is molded from silicone. Hair is implanted into the cap in the various directions naturally grows, giving a natural look. The base can be solid or netted. I have both, and much prefer the netted one, especially in the summer.

Vacuum Fit Base

Also molded, this used to come only in harder matierials such as fiberglass, but now is newly available in a more flexible base. It's the most secure fit you can get, so it's great for people who are very active. The biggest drawback is that it tends to be a bit hot. Since I am not a major athlete and my head tends to get hot easily, I don't have one of these.

Finding a Stylist

The most important thing for any human hair wig is styling. Most wigs need to be thinned and shaped, and the skill required is very different than that of styling growing hair. An experienced wig stylist can give you a cut that makes your hairpiece look like your own hair. An inexperienced one will leave you with hair that has a "wiggy" look that people will recognize a mile away, or worse – even ruin your wig entirely. Once I brought a brand new European hair piece to a wig shop for styling. After settling me and my hair in the chair, the woman unceremoniously grabbed a huge fistful and whacked it off. I ran out the door screaming for help.

One evening a few years ago over a glass of wine, an (ex) boyfriend commented on my hair in a negative way: "Your face is small, and your hair overwhelms your features. Do you know that your wig looks funny in the back? And the color isn't good on you...." At that point I had my wine glass aimed directly at his big fat nose, but then I hesitated. Maybe he was right. I ran to the mirror, and after a long, hard look I had to agree that this hair was just not 'me.' I guess I had grown used to the wiggy look. But my next dilemma was, what was I going to do about it?

The answer came during one of my focus group meetings to gather information for this book. A number of women participated in AA discussions, all with varying degrees of alopecia, in the living room of my home. Some had lost hair and it had grown back. The woman sitting next to me had the most beautiful head of hair and I was so envious. "What lovely hair you have," I said, thinking she was one of the lucky

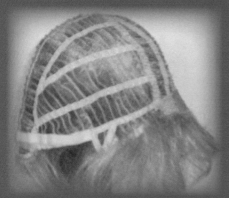

Wefted base

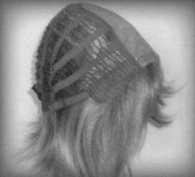

Combination
monofilament
top and wefting

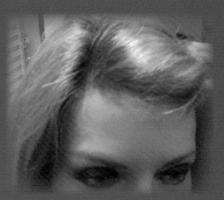

Lace front

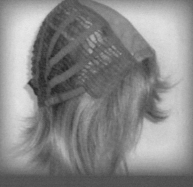

Molded Silicone base
with implanted hair

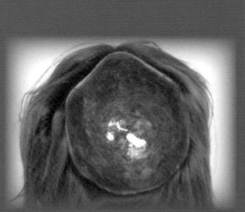

Vacuum fit base

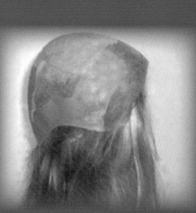

Hand tied

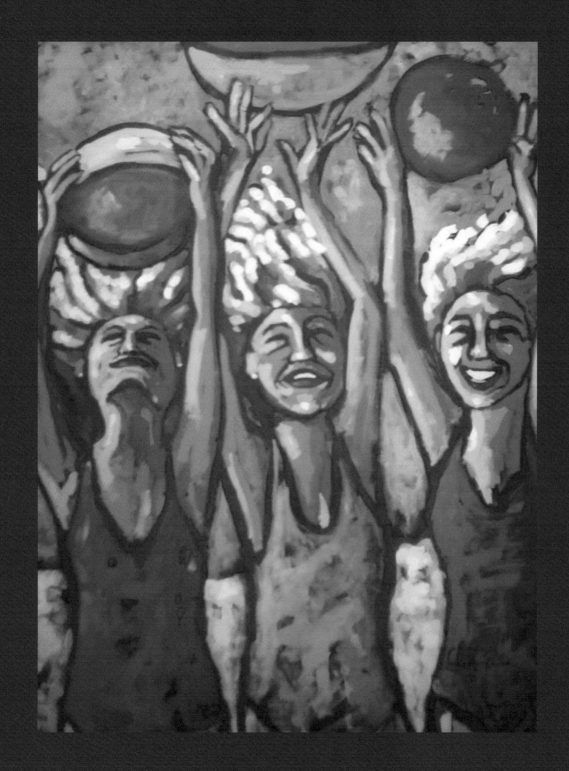

ones who had regrown her hair. "It's a wig," she announced, and proceeded to tell me that she had purchased her yummy locks from Brenda Kay, who also styled them to loook as if they were growing out of her head, right here in Portland.

The next day I was in Brenda's chair and she was measuring me for what turned out to be one of the most beautiful pieces of hair that I had ever seen, let alone put on my head. The body! The texture! The color (like my own, but even better)! And, after she cut and styled my tresses, I have never looked back. (Brenda Kay works with people all over the world, so if you want to contact her see the Resources section.)

Care for Human Hair

Human hair wigs need extra care. Even after my initial cut and style, I still have my stylist keep them up so they continue to look natural and shiny. A hairpiece that is worn daily should be cleaned at least once every three weeks. Or, more often if you notice that your hair is stiff, dull, tangles easily, or clumps up.

If you want to try cleaning and styling your human hair wig yourself, here are a few tips:

1. Fill the sink with water, a squirt of shampoo (I like Biolage), and a tablespoon of baking soda. (Baking soda will cut through the body oils, hair products and dirt better than shampoo alone.)

2. After brushing, immerse your wig for a few seconds, then squeeze the suds through it.

3. Rinse, refill the sink, and add conditioner to the water.

4. Pass the hair through the water briefly, but don't let it soak because that will loosen the hair from the base.

5. Rinse thoroughly and roll in a towel to blot up excess moisture.

6. When the wig is no longer dripping, place it on a canvas block (you can get them at most wig supply stores or catalogs. Be sure you have a size smaller than your actual head so the wig won't stretch out).

7. Using a very wide-toothed comb or pick, comb through the hair. Comb through again, using a finer comb. Comb a third and final time, using a very fine-toothed comb.

8. Don't touch the wig until it has completely dried. If you don't let it dry completely, it will puff out and become stiff and unnatural looking while you are styling.

9. Section off your wig, using clips to hold the uppermost layers. Use a ceramic curling or flat iron to shape your wig. Do two-inch sections at a time from the underside up.

10. Be sure to let your canvas block dry out completely, or it will develop mildew.

11. For curly styles, you can set damp hair on Velcro self-hold rollers (find them at Walgreen's or other variety store).

For Patchy Spots: Partial Wigs, Hair Attachments, Extensions and Scalp Makeup

If you have patchy spots and don't want to go to a full wig but still want coverage, there are some great options:

3/4 Cap Wigs: These sit back on your head so you can pull out your own hair around your forehead and ears and blend them over the top of the wig. Look at Beauty Trends catalogs.

Integration Pieces: Featuring open wefting at the sides and back, you can pull your own hair through openings throughout the wig for a really natural look and have coverage for your spots. You'll find some styles in Paula Young catalogs.

Sleep Wigs: The Wig Company catalog offers wigs you can sleep in that have hair connected to a lace headband. Amy's Presence has a wig they make especially for sleeping.

Attachments: All these catalogs feature ponytails and other attachments that are easy to clip on.

Scalp Makeup:

Many people swear by an application of matte eyeshadow on the bald spots, but there are also some great products on the market made especially for disguising them (even used in Hollywood for actors and models). The best place to find these helpers is online at Folica.com. DermMatch comes in a compact with its own applicator. Wet and apply to the bare skin and pale new hair growth. It will last until the next shampoo, and you can swim with it on. Toppik Hair Building Fibers really help mask the thinning spots. Just shake it on your head and if you want to be extra secure, spritz hairspray on it. It works well over DermMatch, adding texture for a natural effect. There are also several different types of canned spray hair paint. A favorite is Bumble and Bumble colored hair powder spray. This works great along the hairline and can also thicken the appearance of your overall head of hair; just lift the hair in sections and spray.

Hair Extensions:

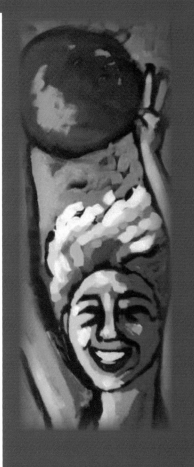

Too bad hair extensions weren't around when I had patchy spots — this is something I would have been very interested in trying. But before you run down to the nearest salon, here are some things you should know.

Hair extensions are lengths of human or synthetic hair attached near your scalp in such a way that it can hide your bald spots. Well done extensions by a skilled stylist will match your hair in color and texture and blend in naturally. Depending on how they are applied, they can be worn anywhere from one day to up to six months.

Types of extensions include clip-ins (falls which are free-hanging hair sewn into netting or ponytails and puffs), strands of up to fifty individual hairs, hand or machine made wefts, or clusters of hair secured at the top and woven into a band, and braids and locks, which are visible but blend into the hairstyle. Amber tells me there are also wefted, skin-based or polyurethane extensions which are affordable, easy on the hair and scalp, and almost impossible to detect.

These different types of extensions are attached in various ways. Clip-in ponytails can be secured with barrettes, falls and wefts are attached with tiny combs. Clip-ins are the easiest on your hair and you can reuse them (I've included a quick and easy lesson on how to apply them below). You might like Hair U Wear's Raquel Welch line. These are human hair and can be colored, flatironed or curled. Also take a look at the Paula Young catalog for reasonably priced human hair clip-ins. There are even extensions you can tape in (J Paul Wrap Around Color Extensions, available from Beauty Trends) and remove easily. The color choices are limited, however.

Wefts are either glued to your scalp with liquid adhesive, or sewn into micro cornrows of your own hair. Strands are fused, or bonded, with pieces of your own hair, using heat or ultrasonic waves; they can also be attached to your own hair with micro-rings, or tiny metal rings.

Be aware that different kinds of hair will give you different looks. For example, I advise you to stay away from synthetic extensions, unless you want to look like you have a shredded plastic bag stuck to your head. They will frizz when you sleep on them, and frizz in the heat. You can't use your blowdryer or curling iron. They may be the least expensive, but they're no bargain. Instead, use human hair that has a similar texture as your own. And speaking of cost, it really varies – anywhere from a few hundred to thousands of dollars. You'll have to locate a good "hair extensionist," and go from there. Ask trusted friends; even your doctor may know. A reputable company to ask about is Great Lengths, which provides hair extensions to many celebrities such as Paris Hilton and Nicole Ritchie, and some of us mortals, too!

Some women with patchy spots swear by hair extensions. "I've been using hair extensions for the past five years with no problems at all," says Caroline, a pediatric nurse. "It's just about where you get them done. Get a recommendation from someone you trust who has hair extensions."

And then again, there are some who have had bad experiences. Says Bonnie, an actress, "I had hair extensions done once. They hurt so much, I had to have them removed after a few days. When they came out, I had more bald spots!"

If it hurts, run. Pulling out more of your hair is not the idea!

Add Your Own Clip-ins

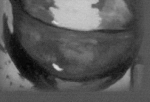

1. Draw a comb horizontally from ear to ear from nape to crown, into two to four sections, about three inches apart.

2. Start at the nape. Tease hair at the roots and lightly spritz with hair spray. Attach the extension as close to your scalp as you can.

3. Repeat with each section.

4. After application, you may need to have someone snip the extensions so they blend into your own hair.

Sleeping with Wigs

I have three inexpensive wigs I use just for sleeping. I mean, what if there's a fire or an earthquake and you have to run out of the house? What if a burglar comes into your bedroom and sees you without a wig (although that is a surefire way to foil a burglary in progress)? Anyway, I choose short and comfy synthetic wigs that won't get in my mouth or eyes, and don't itch. I alternate with soft turbans in colors to match my nighties. They're like little T-shirts for my head. Either way, I can be stylin' as I'm off to dreamland.

Attaching Your Wig

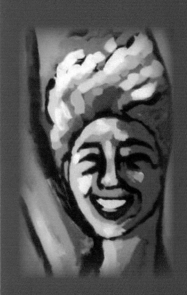

Many synthetics and human hair wigs have netting in the front and top, and double-sided tape (found at wig stores, in catalogs and online) won't work. For these kinds of wigs, I sew small plastic patches at the front, tabs and nape. I use pieces of an old soft plastic shower curtain, but you can also find plasticized fabric in craft stores. There are also 'plasticizing' products you can apply to your wig to create a gripping area for tape or other adhesive. One is called 'Easy Tab' which is available from MHRW International (see Resources section).

My silicone-based wigs are easy to attach with double-sided tape. The custom-fit ones often don't need tape, but I like to attach it just to be secure. Wig tape comes in different strengths, bonding from one to more than thrity days. One good place to find out more about, and order, different types of tape is Hair Direct (see the Resources section for details). Hair Direct also instructs you on how to prepare your scalp for a good bond.

Liquid adhesives are also a popular way to attach your hair system for daily and extended wear. You'll find how-to and purchase information at Hair Direct.

Some women choose to wear their human hair systems 24-7. They wash and wear them just like their own hair. This requires liquid bonding adhesive and a very

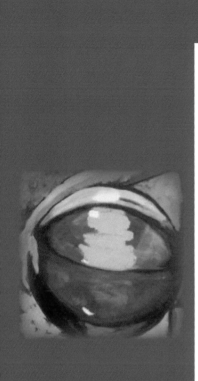

strong bond — the entire unit is glued down to your scalp and stays there until you take it off. Because the glue is strong, taking the wig off carefully is important; otherwise it (and maybe your scalp, too!) could be damaged. Some people have their wigs bonded and removed professionally on a regular basis. I don't think I would want to do this myself — but if you're interested, check with your wig professional to find out more.

If you have patchy spots and are wearing a partial wig or integration piece, simply sew on a small comb (you can usually find packets of them at variety stores or pharmacies) to the middle front. Make a pincurl with bobby pins in your own hair at the hairline and push the comb through. If you have a hairline and want it to show, pull a chunk of your own hair forward over your forehead, and make a pincurl behind it. Attach the piece with the comb, then backcomb or tease your own hair slightly and then smooth it over the hairpiece.

Traveling with Wigs

Synthetics can be great for traveling. You can wash them in a jiffy, they'll dry overnight, and you don't have the hassle of styling. For longer trips, I take along two identical synthetic wigs. When one needs washing, I swish it in the sink and let it dry while I go on my merry way with the other one. (Traveling seems to make hair dirty faster.) However, if you're going to a really hot climate, human hair may be the best solution. I once took a brand new synthetic to Phoenix for a week. As the temperature rose to over a hundred degrees, my wig frizzed into a brillo pad and I couldn't get a brush through it.

It took some humiliating travel experiences to finally learn the wisdom of bringing a backup wig. One was the romantic candlelight dinner experience that turned my hair into a clown wig. Another was when I was on a week-long Caribbean cruise with a girl friend. We were both single and having a dreamy time. I had brought just one wig – a human hair one – and of course with all that fun in the sun it got clumpy and mop-like within a few days. My choices were wear the mop or wash it. Since I was going on a tour of one of the islands the next day with a handsome diving instructor named Bill Beach (wonder if that was his real name?), I decided to wash the mop. After washing it, drying it and trying to curl it back into its original form, I had to accept the fact that the dirty mop

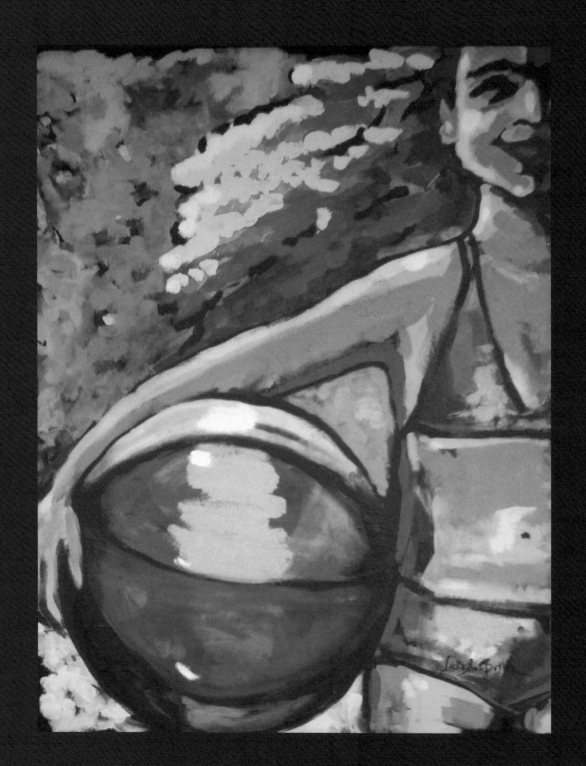

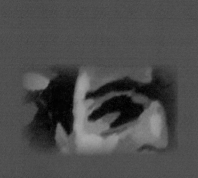

was now an electrified hair ball. And of course, I had to wear it. Bill was nice enough not to ask me about my bad hair day. Maybe he thought that looking like you put your finger in a wall socket was the latest style.

Even when you bring a backup, mishaps can occur. While at a resort in Puerto Vallarta with the aforementioned Rohnn, I shampooed one of my wigs. Wrapping it in a towel to blot out the excess water, I trotted out to the pool in my other wig, and left the first one in the towel on the counter in the bathroom. When we got back after a couple of hours the towel, with the wig in it, was gone, taken by the cleaning staff to the laundry room. With visions of my wig screaming for mercy in a hot dryer, I got on the phone with the cleaning supervisor and shreikingly explained that the drowned animal carcass-like item wrapped in one of the towels was mine, and would they please return it to the room. And yes, I was mortified.

If you travel with human hair, pack tissue into the cavity and place it in a shoebox. This will keep it nicely. For holding your wig at your hotel, some people use a bedpost, but you can't always count on that kind of a bed! I take a fold-up plastic or metal wig stand; they don't take up space in your suitcase. And if you have a wefted wig you can hang it on the robe hook on the bathroom door.

How to Find a Good Wig

Ask around. Ask your dermatologist. Your support group. Check the yellow pages. Go to NAAF.org and click on their "Marketplace." Google "Wigs" online. There are a plethora of resources for wigs today.

If you order a wig on the internet or from a catalog, remember that colors can vary quite a bit from photos to actual hair. Some companies will supply swatches, or sell color rings; or you can send a sample of your own hair for them to match. This is the only way to get the color you like.

Insurance Coverage

In Minnesota and New Hampshire, the law requires insurance carriers, including health maintenance organizations, to cover a "hair prosthesis." Several other states are considering similar legislation. Meanwhile, you may have to convince your insurance company to cover your wig.

If you would like to tackle your insurance carrier, contact NAAF at www.naaf.org and request a packet of information. This will guide you step-by-step, through filing a claim to what to do if your claim is denied. There is also information on how you can help get legislation passed in your state that will mandate insurance coverage for hair prostheses. Amber advises that you state that your 'cranial prosthesis' is for medical reasons. "Your hair is designed to keep you warm, and getting cold often can adversely affect your immune system. Since hats are not always permitted, or socially acceptable, in many places of business, hair is required for your health."

You've Got Style!

It seems obvious that a woman who gets a wig would want it to look as much like her original hair as possible, right? But then again, it's fun to try something different if you're not shy. After all, how many women get a chance to go from short to long and back again, at a moment's notice?

I have yet to figure out what my signature style is, because I enjoy wearing everything from very short to below shoulder length, and curly to straight, depending on my mood. I am – or I should say was – a natural dark blonde, but have various shades of blond wigs, and even a couple of red ones and a black one for my alter ego that I bring out at Halloween. Many Hollywood headliners love the versatility of wigs to change their hairstyle and color from one day to the next – so why not you? Go ahead, pretend you're Britney, Beyoncé or Cher, and have a ball changing your look to fit your mood. While you try new looks, you may discover a wonderful, new and exciting you!

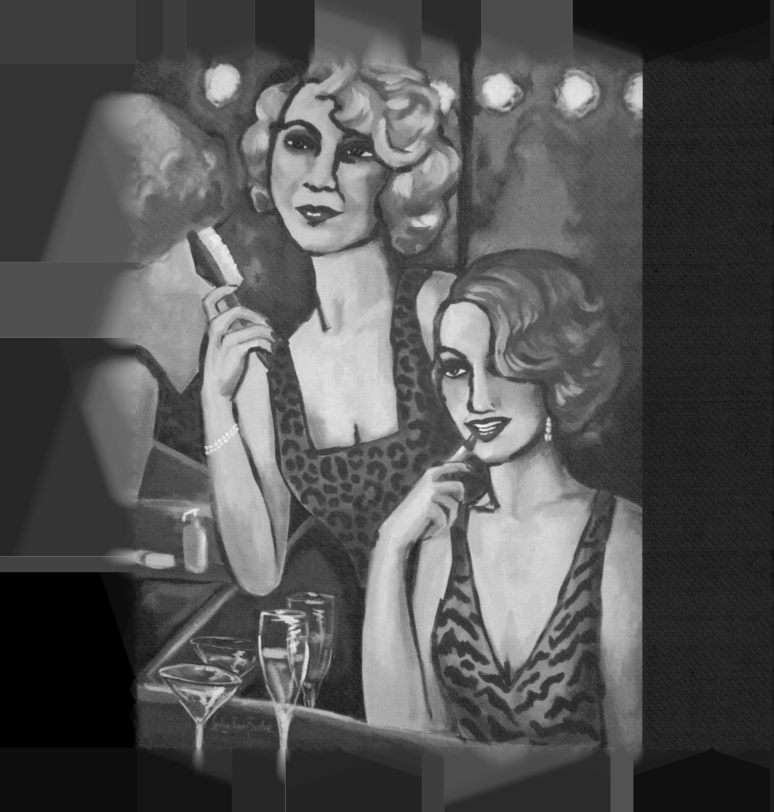

CHAPTER TEN

Get Ready for Your Closeup

Some of us may be fortunate enough to have eyelashes and eyebrows, but if you're like me you're free of fuzz. That means re-learning how to do your makeup.

Eyebrows

The worst eyebrow "do" I ever saw was at an alopecia areata support group several years ago. A pretty, conservatively dressed young woman had painted two black lightning bolts above her eyes. I don't think she meant for them to look like lightning bolts, but she must have thought they were a good substitute for her real eyebrows. I've also seen eyebrows drawn in a single pencil line, shaped in a too-perfect arc, and jotted on to form something similar to slanted exclamation points.

And don't think that professional makeup artists can do it any better. I had a woman make me into a blond version of Joan Crawford.

I also tried some "real hair" eyebrows I ordered from a wig catalog. Although they claimed it was human hair, I think it was actually from a horse. It was stiff and impossible to work with. Then just recently I heard about some synthetic hair eyebrows, and hoping this could be a good product, I sent for them. When I opened the package, I screamed because I thought they had sent me two fuzzy dead worms. I didn't even bother to put them on – just sent them right back. Too thick, too much "hair," too fake looking. If anyone knows the secret to making these real or synthetic hair eyebrows look good, let me know!

Instead I recommend a product called Beauti-Full Brows by J.A.H. Creations, which are "removable tattoo eyebrows." The brows are smudgeproof, waterproof and last for days (on me they will last from one to three days). If you have oily skin like I do, they will wear longer if you prepare your eyebrow area by swabbing it with alcohol (this also removes the old eyebrows). These brows are quite inexpensive. I have to say that it's a little difficult lining them up so they are even on both sides, but like everything else it just takes practice. There are many different styles and colors and it can take several tries to find the right one. I pasted on six different types of eyebrows over a period of several weeks (amazingly, no one seemed to notice). I finally found one the right shape, but it was too light. However Angela, the inventor of these eyebrows, made a new brow in the shape and color I requested.

If you would rather draw on your own brows (remember that they will probably have to be touched up at least once a day), you can learn to make them look natural. I have a bit of an advantage, since I'm an artist and have a knack for faces. So, I'm going to proceed with an eyebrow art class.

Eyebrow Drawing Lesson

1. Dab some face powder on your eyebrow ridge. This will help the drawn-on eyebrows wear longer.

2. With a sharp angled brush (the ones you find in the eyebrow powder compacts are good), apply eyebrow powder or eye shadow in a color close to your natural brows. Use a light, angled sweeping motion to make small strokes close together in the brow shape you want (Bonus! You can create your own shape: more or less arched, and even a little further up on your forehead if your brows have dropped with age). Don't try to make it look exactly like hair, and don't make it too precise.

I never realized until lately that women were supposed to be the inferior sex.

Katharine Hepburn

3. With a freshly sharpened eyebrow pencil, use the same light, feathery motions to draw little hairs on top of the powder. A sweeping motion will make the stroke darker at the "root" and lighter at the end of the "hair" for a more natural look.

You may want to practice several times to get the feel of it. If you've done it correctly, you'll have a pretty good rendition of real eyebrows!

4. Lightly powder over the top of your new eyebrows. And be careful not to rub because they will come off. (This is hard when you wear bangs because either the hairs tickle or your push them out of your eyes – and then you have a blank spot where a few eyebrow hairs used to be. Try not to touch!) I've tried various products that are supposed to seal eyeshadow and pencil (some people swear by hairspray and a product called "Liquid Bandaid"). The best one I've found is called Liner Last eyeliner sealant. It works fairly well, lasting all day if you're careful. It dries shiny so you have to powder it lightly.

5. If you have bangs, wisp them down on your forehead. Your eyebrows, peeking out behind them, will look natural.

Eyelashes

I used to wear false eyelashes all the time (you can find inexpensive ones at most drug stores and many wig shops). However, since they have yet to make a foolproof eyelash glue that will not let you down in the middle of dinner or tears (let alone sweating or swimming!), I wear them only when I know I'm going to be scrupulously examined or am having my photo taken.

I have been tempted to try the semi-permanent eyelash glue for individual eyelashes, but it smells so strong that it makes my eyes water; it might be too hard on eyelid skin. A few years ago, someone mentioned a product called "Diamond" hair bond glue that supposedly is safe and keeps your false eyelashes on for a couple of weeks, but I can't find anyone who carries it. Maybe you'll have better luck.

I have found a pretty safe system for applying them, so you might want to try this. If not, I will also tell you how to make your eyes appear lashed even when you're not wearing any.

What really matters is what you do with what you have.

Shirley Lord, Vogue Editor

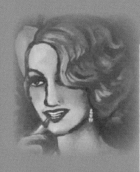

False eyelashes that look good and last longer:

1. Most eyelashes right out of the box are too long and even. Trim them a little bit with cuticle scissors: make them somewhat uneven, and make them shorter by cutting them at the outer corner of the eye. An exception is Ardell, #110 eyelashes. I can plop them right on with no trimming. Another of my favorite styles is Ardell #120. You can get them at most any large variety store, as well as online.

2. I've also found that two pairs of eyelashes worn at the same time often looks more realistic. Wear a pair trimmed shorter as a base, and the second pair trimmed the length you want it.

3. With eyelash glue (I like Ardell brand best, in the dark tone – " clear" goes on white and sometimes stays white in spots. Also, if you're in a hurry it takes too long to disappear) apply a line of glue on the lashes, *and* apply a line across your eyelid where your real eyelashes used to be. I use a toothpick or cocktail pick, or just apply it from the tube. Be careful! And contact lens wearers, don't put your lenses in until after you apply the lashes or you could ruin your contacts.

4. Let the glue dry a little so it's tacky. I use tweezers to place the lashes precisely on the lid, adjust them – push them into your skin a little bit for a good, tight bond – and hold them until they set. Don't bother with the pink curved applicator that you get with eyelash kits, it's useless. Also, don't get too close to the inside of your eye; moisture from your tear duct will loosen the glue.

5. Lower your lids a bit to check for any gaps. You don't want someone to discover that you have a half-on eyelash in the middle of an important moment!

6. With a very small brush or sponge applicator, apply dark brown or black eyeshadow or eyeliner to the lid and over the base of the eyelashes. It will camouflage the glue line. Also, dark-toned glue dries shiny (why did they do that?), cover up that shine so it won't look weird.

7. Smudge the eyeshadow/eyeliner so it's smoky and fades up the lid. You can also use a different color above the dark brown or black base.

8. Finally, apply a light coat of mascara – you will be amazed at how real your eyelashes will look!

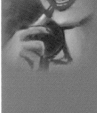

9. Be sure to take your eyelash glue, toothpick and tweezers with you if you're going out so you can fasten down a corner if you need to.

10. Don't get frustrated. It gets easier every time!

11. Cleaning them is easy, too. After taking the lashes off, the glue usually peels right off the lash strip. If there are still clumps of glue, soak the lashes in a little bit of cleaning fluid for a few minutes (in an old plastic vitamin bottle top, I put enough Afta to cover the lashes and let them sit for no more than five minutes). Take them out and put on an old towel, then brush the softened glue out with an old mascara wand or other tiny brush.

12. To get the glue off your eyelids, I've found that Ponds cleansing towelettes work really well. It only takes one or two swipes and it's gentle on your eyes.

Note that there are also false eyelashes available for your lower lids. Follow the same instructions, except just use one set. If you want to wear top lashes only, follow the instructions below for the bottom lids.

No eyelashes that look like you have eyelashes:

This works best when you have long bangs that fall over your eyebrows. The look is right in style for the "smoky eye." Don't be afraid to use the dark eyeshadow – I'm blonde and fair, and I wear this look every day.

1. Apply face powder around the eye area.

2. With a medium to dark-toned eyeshadow, sweep color across your lids and feather up just past the crease. I use different colors: dark gray, amethyst, navy blue or dark brown.

3. With dark (black or very dark brown) eyeliner, outline the entire eye. I use black eyeshadow dipped in water to make it intense. You can use a liquid eyeliner if you like, but it doesn't blend into the shadow as well as the powder, and it usually flakes.

4. Smudge so that the liner and the shadow blend together.

5. Voilà, a smoky eye that looks pretty damn good, even if you don't have eyelashes!

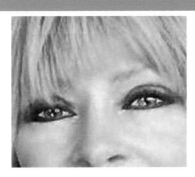

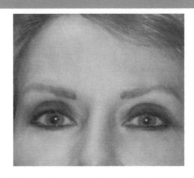

*False eyelashes
and drawn-on eyebrows*

*Eye makeup without false lashes,
and temporary tattoo eyebrows*

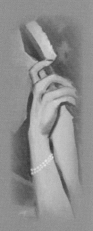

Facial Tattooing

Permanent makeup sounds like a good idea; specialists in cosmetic tattooing can give you little eyebrow "hairs" and eyeliner that won't rub off. I had both procedures done about fifteen years ago. Would I do it again? Absolutely not.

The eyebrow "hair" lines didn't come out as fine as I had hoped. They looked thicker, undefined and continued to spread out until they disappeared, within the space of three years. Now I have a light blue shadow that won't go away that I have to cover up with makeup. You can see it in the photo above. (How it got to be blue, I don't know! As far as I know, the cosmetician was using brown!). Also, I have quite a few scars in my eyebrow area from the procedures. I have never had them redone, because I think the ones I draw on by hand, and the temporary "tattoo" eyebrows, look more natural.

The tattooed eyebrows I have seen on other women just don't look natural. One otherwise beautiful lady had hers done several years ago and now they have a greenish cast. It's so horribly fascinating that, when she talks, I look into her eyebrows instead of her eyes.

The pain of getting tattooed eyeliner rates a number fifteen on a scale of one to ten. Like the eyebrows, eyeliner took several sessions. During one session I felt searing pain, and it hurt so badly and my eyes were watering so much, I could hardly drive home. At the next session, I told the technician I thought she had stuck the needle into my eye. Insulted and waving her needle ominously in my face, she adamantly denied it. Not wanting to experience further excruciating agony, I didn't argue with her! However, at my next eye exam the eye doctor asked me where the black spot had come from. "It looks like ink!" He exclaimed. The final insult: after all this pain and trauma, I have no eyeliner. It faded very quickly (within about a year) and with the threat of more horrific pain, I never went back.

It's the policy of the National Alopecia Areata Foundation not to recommend tattooing for those reasons, and more. It's an invasive procedure, and there are risks. For example, say you have your eyebrows tattooed in one place, and then your hair grows back...in a different place! Also, be aware that certain tattoo ink colors contain iron oxide that consists of real pieces of metal. This can interfere with certain laser procedures and MRIs, causing second-degree burns and blistering. Recently, the FDA issued a warning that certain inks used in the facial tattooing process have caused adverse reactions, such as swelling, cracking, peeling, blistering and scarring.

After all these dire warnings, in all fairness I have to tell you that some women swear by their tattooed eyebrows and eyeliner. If you decide to go ahead, proceed with caution. Make sure that person comes with sterling recommendations and sterile needles, and that they show you their work on other people with your condition.

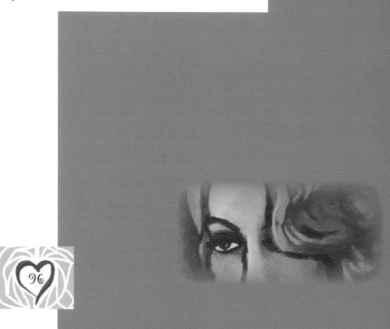

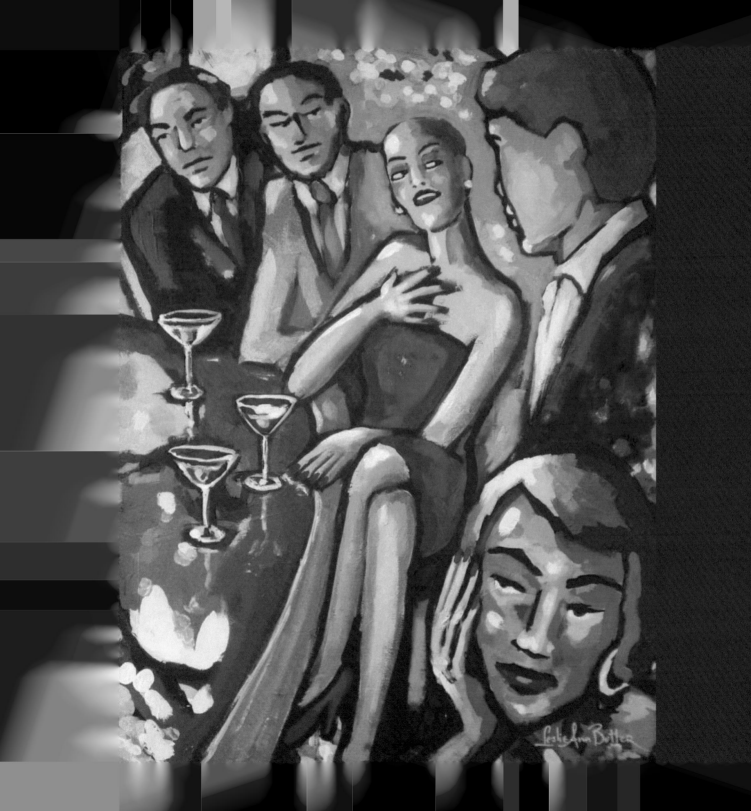

CHAPTER ELEVEN

Getting Your Groove Back

Losing hair on your head and around your eyes can wreak havoc with your feeling of femininity. "Am I still sexy?" you ask yourself. "Am I even attractive?" No matter how many people tell you that you've still "got it," the number one person you have to convince is yourself. And just how are you supposed to do that?

There's no single way. I can tell you what helped me, but if you spend some time curled up with a cup of tea and a pad and paper, you will come up with some of your own ideas about how to get your groove back.

After all my hair fell out I didn't feel very feminine any more. I was afraid to toss my crowning glory, I couldn't bat my (non-existent) eyelashes or arch a hairless brow. But then I suddenly started craving the color pink. I just had to have it; everything from pale peach to soft powdery pink. From my head to my feet, to my underwear. Up till then, I didn't have a single stitch of pink in my wardrobe. But now I had everything from pink lipstick to pink cowboy boots. It made me feel girly. Some people even started to call me Pinky. That and shaking my booty (now the Devil with the Pink Dress) made the world rosier. But it was therapeutic for me; in fact, according to a recent research study, men who were told they would become weaker after viewing the color pink lost strength when tested with grip machines. Women, however, became stronger after viewing the color. So there you have it – Pink Power!

Denise, forty-four, a software specialist tells her secret: "I became a blonde. I always had mousey-colored hair. But when I finally had to start wearing wigs, I chose streaky blonde. To be perfectly honest, the wig flattered me and looked better than my own hair ever had! I felt sexier! And men paid more attention to me."

Marilyn, forty, a store owner says: "At first I thought I was never going to attract a man again. Recently divorced, I thought I'd always be single, and I didn't even try to look good. But then at an AA support group I noticed a lovely woman who was about my age. She was bald, wearing a wig, and she looked dynamite! It made me realize I had to get back to living my life in a normal, healthy way. A few days later I had a facial, got a free makeup consultation at a department store, bought myself a new outfit and got a more flattering wig. Look out, world!"

Julia, twenty-nine, an airline attendant, says: "I went into a deep depression for awhile and had to go to counseling. That helped, but I still didn't feel good enough, or that I was "whole." And I was lonely. What really did help me was getting my cat from the local shelter. Clyde needed me. And he ended up being just what *I* needed! His unconditional love worked its way into my heart and made me realize that I was good, whole and beautiful just the way I was, and that I didn't have to feel defective just because of AA. Clyde was the factor that made me get up and look people in the eye again, and feel good about myself! A few months later, my new attitude attracted this wonderful man, who is now my husband. And of course, he loves Clyde!"

"You have to accept yourself the way you are without hair," says Natalie, twenty-two. "At first I tried to wish it away, cry it away, drink it away! Finally I just had to deal with it. I got a wig that made me look pretty damn good, and I signed up for a class in modeling. I learned how to walk beautifully – glide, glide, glide – I still hear that ringing in my ears, even when I'm in my sweats and tennis athletic shoes! I realize I had been clumping around hunched over, trying to fly under the radar. I learned more about makeup, too. Now when I go down the street I see my reflection in store windows and feel like I'm grace personified! It makes me feel very confident. I get lots of appreciative looks, too!"

Love is a great beautifier.

Louisa May Alcott, Novelist

People driving past and guys in clubs will always look at long hair and your ass.
Nicola Charles, Actress

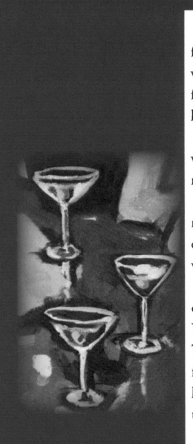

Adele, a forty-five-year-old manager, confesses she had cosmetic surgery. "I had fake eyebrows, false eyelashes, fake hair, so I thought, *What the heck,* I'd just go for the whole plastic thing and get a facelift and boob job! I have to tell you that it made me feel like a million dollars. The only downside is that I have scars on my head – with no hair to cover them. Guess I'm not going bareheaded anymore!"

Paige told me that her salvation was yoga. "The spiritual mind-body connection was exactly what I needed. I can't tell you how much it changed the way I feel about myself."

"Prayer and meditation helped me," says Jane, a nurse. "At first, I just prayed for my hair to grow back. But later, I realized that what I needed to pray for and meditate on was strength to handle whatever happens. We may not always get what we want, but we get what we need. This knowledge has given me peace and self-acceptance."

Laura, who has had alopecia since she was thirteen, says: "The thing I would tell other women who are attempting to deal with this is, stop trying to figure out 'why.' You will drive yourself crazy! My advice would be to just accept and surrender to it. There is so much peace with acceptance! That, and start wearing a wig sooner. I waited for two years while my hair got patchier and thinner and the whole time I was thinking how hideous I looked. But the minute I accepted it and put on that wig, I felt a million times better. I could have saved myself two years of misery if I had only known!"

There are many other large and small things that can help you feel like *you* again. You have to decide what they are, and give yourself permission to do them. It's perfectly all right to indulge yourself, so that you can get back on course – or forge yourself a new one. By stepping out, you may discover your own magic that will help you surpass anything you've done before. Many women report that they get to a point where they feel many times better about themselves than they did when they had all that hair.

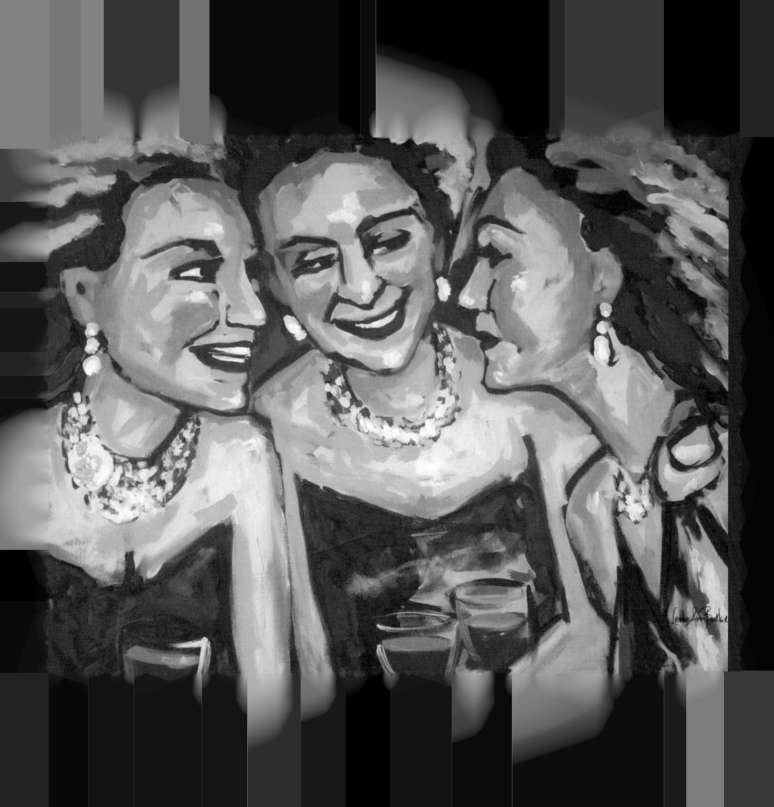

CHAPTER TWELVE

No Bad Hair Days

When my friends complain about their bad hair days, I just tell them that whenever I have one I take my hair off and put on a different wig!

Whether you have hair in patches, wear wigs, or are bald, the most attractive thing you can do is be comfortable with yourself. Decide that alopecia is not going to impact your life in a negative way.

Every day, when you put on your wig, or your spot coverup, your hat, your false eyelashes, don an attitude as well. It may not feel natural at first, but when you walk into a room, try saying to yourself something like this: "I am sexy/attractive/popular! Everyone loves me and I feel the same about them!" (Practice at home first. Carry a card in your purse or pocket to look at as a reminder.) Changing your attitude will also change your perception of yourself and others. You might have to fake it at first. Become an actor. I took theater in high school to overcome my shyness. I enjoyed it so much, I majored in theater in college. Now I can hardly remember how it feels to be shy. If you do it again and again, it becomes real. Eventually, you will feel like the most attractive person in the room – and you just may be!

> I'd rather be bald on top than bald inside.
>
> *Joe Garagiola*

I have a friend named Carole who embodies that philosophy. She is as cute as a button, with hair the color of burnished mahogany. The first thing you notice isn't her thin hair (she had patchy bald areas) – it's her smile and her eyes. When she walks into a room, people flock to her. Carole doesn't worry about how she appears. She concentrates on others. She asks about them, she listens, she cares. She generates a beam of love that everyone picks up on. That makes her beautiful.

As Ronald D. Bissell, author of *Reflections: Mirrors of Light* said, "It is every moment of your life that forms the river you travel. Whether the moments are easy or difficult, they add together to form something beautiful – they form who you are."

Don't be afraid to be who you are; allow your experiences to help you grow and embrace life rather than be fearful.

With your new crowning glory, walk into your office, the gym, a restaurant or a party with a big grin on your face. Ask your friends how they like it, and ask them if they think you should get streaks or go lighter or darker. Make it fun for them. Let any thoughts of 'poor me' fade away with yesterday's tears and fears. With this attitude, you will become happier and more beautiful than ever before. Believe it. And so will everyone else.

Alopecia can humble you. It can make you cry. It can show you who your true friends are and what kind of stuff your husband is made of. And it can make you strong, kind and wise. I think about the saying, "If it doesn't kill you, it will make you stronger." Alopecia areata is certainly not going to kill you. That leaves you with the only other option.

103

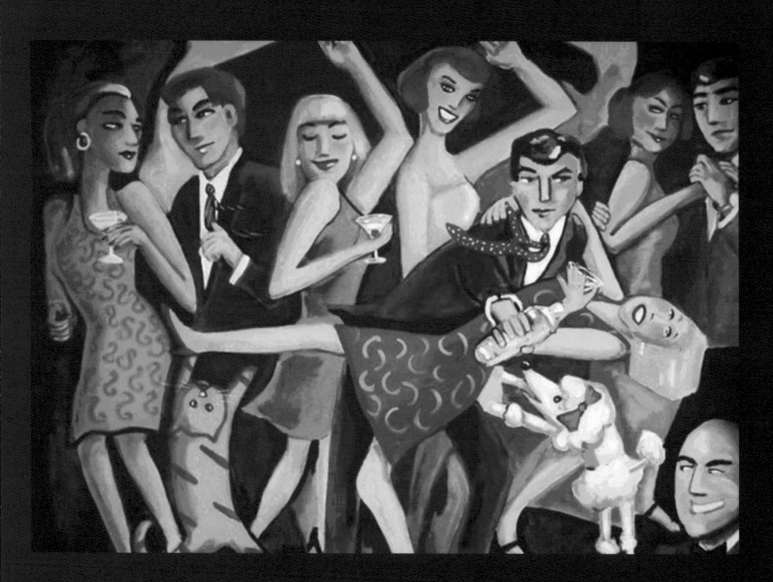

CHAPTER THIRTEEN

Last Thoughts Off the Top of My Head

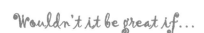

Wouldn't it be great if...

— A bald woman was on the cover of Vogue, and being hairless became the ultimate in stylishness. Think Egyptian queens!

— *All* the celebrities who have experienced any form of AA would come forward with their stories and support.

— Those people who make fun of your baldness or make you uncomfortable in any way lost their hair at that very instant.

— Mascara became unfashionable because the new look was *no* eyelashes.

— People looked on the outside like they are on the inside.

— Kids never got AA.

Products I'd Like to See (is anyone listening?):

– Pre-made wigs that come with a little plastic piece in the front so you don't have to sew one in yourself.

– Dulling spray to make synthetic wigs look natural. (Better yet, synthetic wigs that don't have that fakey shine in the first place!)

– Eyelash glue that's *really* waterproof.

– Hair eyebrows that are soft and natural, easy to work with, and affordable.

Don't you just hate it when...

– People want to feel your wig or look under the edges.

– The man in your life avoids touching your hair.

– A friend says how great it must be not to have to do your hair, and wigs must be so much fun.

– You're trying on clothes in a store dressing room and when you pull something over your head your hair comes off.

– You have no hair on your head, but you have hair on your toes and knuckles.

– People ask if you have pubic hair.

– Your wig starts to itch and all you want to do is rip it off, but you're in a meeting.

– You decide it's time to tell your girlfriends that you have alopecia and wear wigs, and they already know about it.

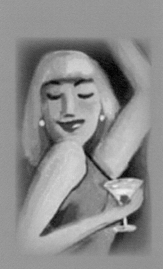

– Out of the corner of your eye you see your dog lying on the floor and start cooing baby-talk to him, then notice it's your wig instead.

– People tell you your wig looks better than your real hair did.

– You accidentally leave a wig lying around when the handyman comes over and he screams when he sees it.

And the good news is:

– You don't have to shave your legs or have a bikini wax.

– Having a bad hair day? Put on a different wig, or don't wear anything.

– If you're at a dull party, you can liven things up by pulling off your wig and tossing it in the chip dip.

– Awareness for this condition is much more prevalent than it was ten years ago.

– You can be blonde one day, brunette the next, and redhead the day after that, and go from short to long to short again.

– If a bear (or an ex-boyfriend) comes in and grabs you by the hair, it's easy to get away.

– You're on the right track to be an Olympic swimmer.

– You can try out for the L.A. Lakers.

– If a pigeon poops on your head, it's a lot easier to clean up.

– Skin without hair feels like velvet.

– Research to find a cure for alopecia areata is being done as you read this.

I loved having a shaved head...

Natalie Portman, Actress, regarding a requirement for a role

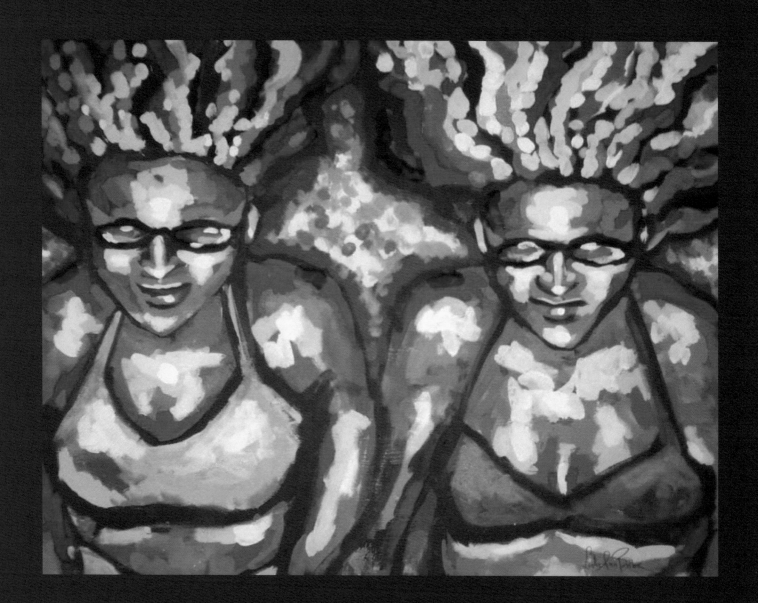

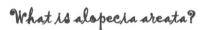

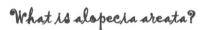

CHAPTER FOURTEEN

Frequently Asked Questions

What is alopecia areata?

Alopecia areata is the umbrella term used to describe patchy hair loss, total scalp hair loss (alopecia totalis), and complete scalp, facial and body hair loss (alopecia universalis). It occurs in males and females of all ages, but onset most often begins in childhood.

How common is it?

It's fairly common. Nearly five million people in the United States have alopecia areata.

Is it hereditary?

Yes, heredity can be a factor in alopecia. In one out of five cases of alopecia, someone else in the family has it. There is a 7% chance you will pass it on to your children.

What triggers alopecia?

It's not known why alopecia starts, or whether it comes from an external source, like a virus, or internally. Research points to genetics.

Will my hair grow back?

Your hair can regrow completely even after years of extensive hair loss. It can also fall out again.

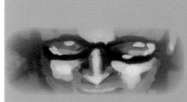

Is alopecia areata caused by stress?

Stress has not been shown to cause alopecia.

Is there a cure for alopecia areata?

At this writing there is no cure. Extensive worldwide research is being done to find the cause and treatment for all forms of alopecia areata.

What treatments area available?

For patchy baldness there are cortisone injections, topical minoxidil, and anthralin cream. For extensive alopecia there are cortisone pills, minoxidil, and topical immunotherapy. The treatments are effective in milder cases, but none are universally effective.

How do I find a support group?

Ask your doctor, or find a support group in your area through NAAF. There are groups all over the world as well as telephone support contacts.

How do I find a good wig?

The NAAF marketplace is a good place to start. Go to their web site and click on "Marketplace." There are links to several good wig companies. And 10% of your purchase goes to benefit NAAF. There are also catalogs and other online sites. The best thing, of course, is to try them on. Your doctor should be able to give you recommendations of wig suppliers in your city.

How about wigs for children?

In the Resources section, you will find several suggestions for finding children's wigs, including Locks of Love and Wigs for Kids, non-profit organizations that provide hairpieces to financially disadvantaged children eighteen years and younger.

Are there any famous people who have alopecia areata?

Yes, some we know about for sure, and some we can only surmise.

Christopher Reeve had alopecia totalis. Princess Caroline of Monaco briefly had it in 1995. Neve Campbell, Whoopi Goldberg, Roger Maris, Humphrey Bogart, John D. Rockefeller, Queen Elizabeth and the Mona Lisa are others who have been named as possibly having alopecia areata. In regards to the historical ladies named, apparently in bygone centuries eyebrow and eyelash plucking was in vogue – maybe it will come back in style again!

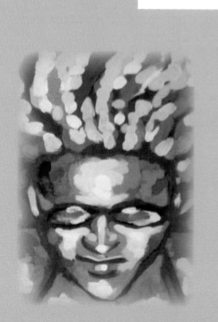

Resources

General Information:

Alopecia World
A social networking site; free membership.
www.alopeciaworld.com

National Alopecia Areata Foundation
PO Box 150760
San Rafael, CA 94915-0760
Phone 415-472-3780
Fax 415-472-5343
info@naaf.org
www.naaf.org

North America Hair Research Society
Website: www.nahrs.org

American Hair Loss Association
www.americanhairloss.org

Dr. Janet Roberts, Dermatologist
2330 NW Flanders St. Suite 201
Portland, OR 97210
503-223-1933

Alopecia Areata, Understanding and Coping with Hair Loss
By Wendy Thompson, M.A. and Jerry Shapiro, M.D.
Published by Johns Hopkins University Press

Manuel Casanova, M.D.
Department of Psychiatry
University of Louisville
500 S Preston St. Bldg 55A, Suite 210
Louisville, KY 40202
502-852-4077

Synthetic and Human Hair Wigs, Consultation and Styling:

Brenda Kay Hair Specialties
1975 SW First Avenue, Suite A
Portland, OR 97201
503-223-8092
www.brendakayhairspecialties.com

Amy's Presence
Crown and Glory Enterprises
www.amyspresence.com

Amber Humphrey
Amber's Anointed Touch Hair Replacement
3915 NW Sitka Place
Corvallis, OR 97330
Phone: 541-752-1444 or 1-800-290-2201
Fax: 541-757-9040
www.Ambersintegrityhairreplacement.com

Vacuum-Based Wigs

Brenda Kay Hair Specialties
See *Synthetic and Human Hair Wigs* for contact information

Peggy Knight Solutions, Inc
180 Harbor Dr., Suite 221
Sausalito, CA 94965
Phone: 415-289-1777 or 800-997-7753
www.peggyknight.com

New Hair Technology
65 West 55th Street, 4th Floor
New York, NY 10019
Phone: 212-581-5900 or 800-434-4552
Fax: 212-265-5652
www.nuhair.com

Styles for African American women:

Wigs by Paula Young
P.O. Box 483
Brockton, MA 02303
1-800-343-9695
www.paulayoung.com

Especially Yours Quality Wigs and Apparel
P.O. Box 105
South Easton, MA 02375
1-800-939-9447
www.EspeciallyYours.com

Hair Addition
888-947-9447
www.hairaddition.com

ILUVWIGS
1-800-966-4079
www.iluvwigs.com

Wigland
1101 NE Broadway
Portland, OR 97232
503-282-1664

Major Brand Wigs Online at a Discount:

Wig Salon.Com Online Catalog
www.wigsalon.com

Feke Wigs
Fekewigs.com

Lori's Wigsite
www.loriswigsite.com

The Wig Mall
www.thewigmall.com

Inexpensive Synthetic Wigs and Attachments:

Wigs by Paula Young
See *Styles for African American Women*
For contact information

Beauty Trends
P.O. Box 9323
Hialeah, FL 33014-9323
1-800-777-7772
www.BeautyTrends.com

The Wig Company
P.O. Box 12950
Pittsburgh, PA 15241-0950
1-800-444-1788
www.twcwigs.com

Headcovers Unlimited
35B Tiffany Plaza
Ardmore, OK 73401
580-226-5871
www.Headcovers.com

Children's Wigs:

Headcovers Unlimited
See *Inexpensive Synthetic Wigs* for contact information

New Hair Technology
See *Vacuum-Based Wigs* for contact information

Locks of Love
2925 10th Ave N., Suite 102
Lake Worth, FL 33461
888-896-1588
www.locksoflove.org

Wigs for Kids
440-333-4433
www.wigsforkids.org

Angel Hair Foundation
2783 Suncrest Avenue
Eugene, OR 97405
541-344-5135
www.angelhairfoundation.org

Hats and Other Head Coverings:

Headcovers Unlimited
See *Inexpensive Synthetic Wigs* for contact information

Just in Time
P.O. Box 27693
Philadelphia, PA 19118
215-247-8777
www.softhats.com

Temporary "Tattoo" Eyebrows:

Beauti-Full-Brows
J.A.H Creations
71 Westervelt Place
Teaneck, NJ 07666
800-241-1598
www.beauti-fullBrows.com

Make Your Own Wigs:

Men's Hair Replacement Workshop
(For women too)
1-866-685-8382
www.MHRW.com

Scalp Makeup (Hair Loss Concealer):

Folica, Inc.
8 Corporate Drive
Cranbury, N.J. 08512
888-919-4247
www.folica.com

Makeup and Styling Tips:

Look Good, Feel Better
1-800-395-LOOK
www.lookgoodfeelbetter.org

Eyebrow Makeup Sealant:

Liner Last ™
EI Solutions
www.eisolutions365.com

Bonding Adhesives: Tape and Liquid:

Hair Direct
800-424-7346
www.hairdirect.com

MHRW International
866-685-8382
www.MHRW.com

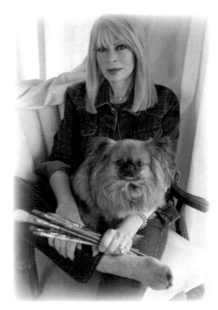

LeslieAnn and Huey

LeslieAnn Butler, artist, author of two books, and former writer and creative director for multi-national advertising agencies in San Francisco and Portland, and former photography and runway model, has won numerous regional and national awards for creativity.

The paintings LeslieAnn used to illustrate this book were chosen from a body of work that has developed over a course of twelve years. As her style has evolved, her newer work features a looser quality. Many of the paintings used to illustrate this book are available for sale. To find out more, go to LeslieAnn's gallery web site, LAButlerArtist.com.

LeslieAnn is involved in several charitable organizations, and has served on the board of the Oregon Humane Society for the past eight years. A portion of the sales of this book will go to to the National Alopecia Areata Foundation.

Her first book, The Dream Road and Other Tales of Hidden Hills, was the recipient of the National Visionary Award in 1998. A collection of children's stories, it is available on her commissions website, Leslieannbutler.com.

Paintings by LeslieAnn Butler

CPSIA information can be obtained
at www.ICGtesting.com
Printed in the USA
276679LV00002B